W9-DAL-964

.

PUBLIC HEALTH PAPERS

No. 60

THE MEDICAL ASSISTANT:
AN INTERMEDIATE LEVEL OF HEALTH CARE PERSONNEL

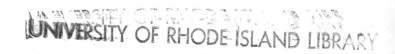

THE
MEDICAL ASSISTANT

An Intermediate Level of Health Care Personnel

Proceedings of an International Conference sponsored by the

John E. Fogarty International Center for Advanced Study in the Health
Sciences, National Institutes of Health, Bethesda, Md, USA

and the

World Health Organization, Geneva, Switzerland,

National Institutes of Health, Bethesda, Md, USA
June 5–7, 1973

Edited by

DONALD M. PITCAIRN, M.D.
Special Assistant to the Director,
Fogarty International Center,
National Institutes of Health,
Bethesda, Md, USA

DANIEL FLAHAULT, M.D.
Chief Medical Officer for Training of
Auxiliary Personnel, Division of Health
Manpower Development, World Health
Organization, Geneva, Switzerland

WORLD HEALTH ORGANIZATION
GENEVA
1974

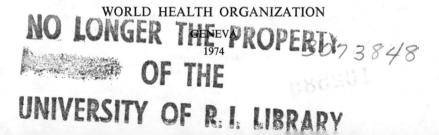

ISBN 92 4 130060 4

PRINTED IN SWITZERLAND

CONTENTS

PREFACE

The medical assistant and other types of intermediate level health personnel are being used in an increasing number of countries to extend the availability of health care and to provide health services in areas where they did not previously exist. The functions that such personnel can perform, their status and the training they should receive are questions of great interest to governments, health authorities, schools providing education in the health sciences, and medical, nursing and other professional bodies.

The John E. Fogarty International Center for Advanced Study in the Health Sciences and the World Health Organization jointly sponsored a three-day conference on this subject in June 1973 at the National Institutes of Health, Bethesda, Maryland. It was believed that a useful purpose would be served by inviting representatives of selected developing countries to meet with people who are engaged in programmes to train auxiliary health personnel in the USA. The participation of people from developing countries was thought desirable, not only because such countries have a long and varied experience with health auxiliaries, but also because their use of medical assistants, in some form, appears to provide a feasible alternative to the production of large numbers of physicians.

There was close cooperation between the Fogarty International Center and the World Health Organization at all stages in the planning and organization of the Conference. The World Health Organization selected a number of countries according to their interest in providing primary health care services through the use of medical assistants, the extent of development of their health services and their geographical distribution. After appropriate consultation, the Fogarty International Center selected participants from the USA whose interests and experience were judged to be most pertinent to the emphasis and purposes of the Conference. Both organizations agreed that attendance should be limited in order to facilitate the free exchange of information.

The concept of the medical assistant is still evolving and will continue to be a subject of debate. The papers presented at the Conference, the statements made and summaries of the discussions have been brought together

7

in this volume which should prove of value to all those concerned in training this type of health personnel and in its use to broaden the scope of basic medical and health services in all countries.

———

INTRODUCTION

by MILO D. LEAVITT, Jr, M.D.[1]

This Conference arose from a series of discussions in 1972 between staff members of the Fogarty International Center and the World Health Organization. The Fogarty International Center was established approximately five years ago. This meeting is precisely the kind of activity the Center was established to undertake; it has brought together here at the National Institutes of Health leading authorities from all over the world to assist us in discussing important problems not only in the biomedical sciences but also in medical education and the provision of health services.

The Conference affords an opportunity to acquaint visiting colleagues with current training programmes in the USA and their future prospects, to compare the USA experience with that in their own countries, and to consider those aspects of training and utilization which might be mutually applicable or beneficial for improving the availability and quality of health services. The recent proliferation of training programmes in the USA underscores the need to examine and clarify such issues as the definition, training, certification and uses of medical assistants.

Some may question the emphasis given to the review of the USA experience. Without some awareness of the complexities of American health care, those who come from less affluent and less technologically advanced countries may not understand the interest taken in the USA in medical assistant programmes. Despite differences between the developed and developing countries, there are many common problems in the provision of health care services, particularly in rural or remote areas. The USA, like many countries, has not yet solved the problems of estimating its health manpower needs or of the best use and distribution of health manpower.

I am very pleased this morning to be able to bring to this group a man who has recently assumed increasing responsibilities at the World Health Organization preparatory to becoming the next Director-General on 21 July 1973. Dr Mahler's presence here this morning was unexpected, but we are grateful that his busy schedule has permitted this opportunity. I am, indeed, very pleased to introduce Dr Mahler.

[1] Director, Fogarty International Center, National Institutes of Health, Bethesda, Md, USA.

ADDRESS

by HALFDAN MAHLER, M.D.[1]

Thank you very much for giving me an opportunity to address your conference. I am as yet only the Director-General elect of WHO and am not due to take up my new duties for several weeks. Thus, I shall speak to you very freely.

There are two subjects which I consider to be the most dramatic of all those with which we have to grapple in medical care. Unfortunately, we seem to be grappling with them in a rather dishonest way and continuing to suggest what we consider to be very clever solutions. It is undeniable that there are important health problems, that some inexpensive technologies are available, and that one can train auxiliaries at low cost to provide some level of health care to millions and millions of people who are totally without health services.

We in WHO have been repeating this for the last twenty years. Many health workers in specific disease fields have been able to standardize certain technologies and lower their cost to about one-thousandth of their current cost in affluent countries—such as the USA and my own. Nevertheless, in the countries whose governments we have tried to assist in translating these technologies into action for the benefit of the health care consumer, very little indeed has happened over the past twenty years.

I, therefore, do not consider over-dramatized a statement of the Executive Board of WHO, contained in an organizational study it made at its January 1973 session, to the effect that the average health care consumer is receiving less care in 1973 than he received 25 years ago when WHO was created. That dramatic statement leaves aside, of course, numerous spectacular achievements, such as the increased average life expectancy. But what good is an increased average life expectancy when an individual cannot receive a reasonable amount of care during those additional years of survival?

This, I think, is the most dramatic fact of all. To underscore that, one need only ask: 'Is there any country today where, if you were given total control over all the resources available for medical care, including political

---

[1] Director-General elect of the World Health Organization, Geneva, Switzerland.

control and control at the most peripheral level, you could not provide a reasonable measure of care to the remotest health care consumer?' The answer, I think, would be that there is no such country.

This is a dramatic fact because, if there were a true conflict between health problems and the cost of health technologies necessary to meet these problems for all consumers, then we would have the right to believe with reasonable honesty that we are trying to do our best, but that the real difficulty lies in lack of funds.

But I do not think that this is true. I am convinced that if you take any field of health technology and bring together the most eminent people in that field, and ask them: 'Which technology is most effective in coping with 90% of a particular health problem in your field?'—I believe in most cases that the reply would be similar to that in my own field, tuberculosis, where it was shown that with only about 2% to 3% of conventional medical technology, we could arrive at roughly 90% of a necessary quality of care. In other words, it is possible to standardize a tiny fraction of a given medical technology so that one can train a health assistant within a relatively short time to provide health care corresponding roughly to the care delivered by a professor or specialist who has had 15 or 20 years of training.

In speaking about tuberculosis I can support my statements by proofs, and I will not venture into other fields, although I have reason to believe that the concept applies. Recently I asked a professor of dermatology, who is an outstanding international expert: 'What do you really have to know in dermatology today to cope with 90% of dermatological problems?' He replied: 'If you know five or six classifications and only a few important kinds of remedies, it is more than enough. What good is it to be able to recognize dermatological diseases if you cannot do something about them? It is only worth while to recognize those conditions that you can treat.' The old management information system theory is still valid: do not collect information if you cannot make use of it. And he added: 'I should think on the whole it would take a week to train somebody to do a respectable job in dermatology.' But people in my country, for example, train for seven or eight years to become respectable members of the dermatological specialty.

When you examine most of the health fields one by one, and you consider the conventional medical knowledge, you discover that you can discard much, leaving only the truly significant medical technology. You also see that you can reduce it with such sharpness of description as to make it possible to train, not a super physician or a super public health nurse, but anyone with a reasonable amount of intelligence and schooling who, if employed in an adequately managed health care system, will deliver exactly the care that he has been taught.

There is nothing new in that. I am sure it is precisely this type of problem which you will be discussing. One must ask the painful question: 'Since there is nothing new in these thoughts, since all of us have been provocative about this matter for years and years and years, why then do things not change?'

We have to say, as a well-known statesman said, that it is infinitely easier to pursue existing policies, even when their failure has become quite evident, than to admit failure and to change the policies. We have to realize that we are all victims of this kind of situation. The most difficult task is to make radical reforms. In other words, the past is our most formidable constraint.

Permit me to give you an example of what I mean. Recently, a very powerful president of a developing country asked me:

'What do you think about the health care system? And I want your personal opinion rather than your view as an official of WHO.'

I replied: 'Sir, I do not think you have a problem because you do not have a health care system.'

He was surprised. 'What do you mean by that?'

'Well, sir, when you consider how the so-called health care system is functioning, you must realize that it is really not functioning. There is a total breach of confidence between the system and the health care consumers who bypass the system, including the hospitals.'

Then he said: 'Well, that is all very well, but what do you think one should do about it?'

I replied: 'I know that you have some excellent people who have been trying to patch up the system for the last few years, but it seems no change has taken place. So, my personal opinion is that you will have to do something much more drastic. But since I am not sure how long you will remain a president, it is for you to decide whether you want to take drastic steps. I think the first step is to close the medical schools for two years. Then we can discuss what the medical schools were supposed to do, because they really constitute the main focus of resistance to change. They speak nicely about introducing reforms, but they are all basically resisting the kind of radical educational reform which is required to make your system function.'

This is a painful indictment for all of us in the health professions. Many of us tend to say that it is the politicians who do not want change. That is not at all true. All presidents or prime ministers today are speaking about revolutionary social reforms required to make the health care system efficient. If we in the health professions were sufficiently courageous and imaginative to suggest to them the necessary solutions, I am sure the aim could be achieved. But we all belong to our own little worlds of entrenched and vested interests, and we seem unable to overcome all the factions within the health professions in order to develop valid political solutions. I do not think you can put the blame on politicians in the conventional sense, not even on the top level politicians. But among the politicians within the health professions, there is something basically wrong.

We should remember to search within ourselves for the true barriers to all the radical reforms which would enable the health assistant to become an effective agent. Simply training millions of health assistants will not help. I have been working in a number of countries where hundreds of thousands of such workers have been trained but are not working efficiently because of an unsuitable health delivery system. No real progress can be made in such a situation. A trained health assistant, unless he is employed within an adequate delivery system, is only a tactical or political excuse. The superficial appearance of accomplishment may conceal its true absence. In one sense, it would be better not to train health assistants if the politician gains the false impression that something positive is being achieved.

Having said this, I readily acknowledge that I am not a magician ready to produce all kinds of solutions. But I fear that grappling with the problem of the health assistant is pointless unless you identify and solve the crude underlying problems.

The same applies, even more dramatically, to the physician. We speak in favour of the community-oriented physician, and many of us in the last 25 years have promoted this concept and have tried to influence the medical curriculum in that direction. I would love to see the country where such community-oriented physicians behave as we want them to behave—that is, organizing a programme and a plan of work for the health team under their control. I do not know if such a country exists, but I would be delighted to visit it for it would give me a good deal of confidence and optimism for the future.

But again, this type of physician will not be able to function efficiently unless certain conditions are fulfilled. In the field of tuberculosis, we did attempt to train not simply chest clinicians but managerial physicians who, with their tuberculosis control teams, should have been able to carry out precisely such community-oriented tasks. We trained them in accordance with the best modern mangerial theories and drew up manuals indicating in detail their daily tasks. We thought we had succeeded and our conscience was relieved. Alas, after their six months of special training, these physicians returned to a system unsuited to them in which they could not operate efficiently or effectively.

If I have any message for you, it is my deep conviction that we must explore and identify more precisely the various categories of health personnel we need in order to give adequate health care at a reasonable price not only to a few people but to all. It is precisely in matters relating to health personnel that we perhaps stand the greatest chance of eventually influencing and assisting the politicians. I am certain that each time we attempt to define the capabilities and potentialities of the medical assistant, we undermine somewhat the existing vested interests and push the front of our attack just a little further. We must be willing to admit that skills are not given by God only to the physician or to the public health nurse; skills can be taught to virtually anyone to meet local conditions and needs. One should be absolutely honest as to who should be trained and what should be taught, and this should not depend upon what degrees or titles follow one's name.

Therefore, I think that whenever you have a group of highly competent people, like those gathered here today, struggling with this kind of problem and expressing their conviction that there is absolutely no reason why we should not have a much better type of care delivery than we have today—each time this happens, you are shaking traditional wisdom, and each time you shake traditional wisdom, the world moves forward.

I believe it is important to recognize that nothing of this sort will be achieved unless radical educational reforms are introduced throughout the system from elementary schooling up through the university. These basic reforms can only come about if we exert continuous pressure on those responsible not only for the final decisions but also for actually implementing them. Each time groups such as this are able to give WHO the ammunition at the right political level to press for such reforms, we take a little step in the right direction.

But it is very hard indeed to keep one's patience, knowing that with appropriate utilization of our skills and resources, everyone today could receive good health care. One can only try to be rational in an irrational world. We must continue to compromise because, after all, we are not presidents and prime ministers of the countries where this ought to be done. This applies not only to developing countries, but also to many developed countries, where superb health care could be provided to everybody at a cost equal, I would say, to roughly one-third or one-fourth of present per capita health care expenditure. Present costs can be afforded in affluent countries where waste seems to be unimportant, but the affluent countries are not my main concern, because they have the funds enabling them to make mistakes, and misery there is not so great or pervasive. The example of the affluent countries is important, however, in that it can contaminate countries which cannot afford that kind of waste.

Therefore, we will not solve this problem unless some very radical changes occur first in the affluent countries and unless we dispel the false notion that medical assistants and other auxiliaries are there to deliver second-rate medical care.

In tuberculosis the auxiliary who has been well trained in specific diagnostic and therapeutic standardized techniques has done much better than the physician who may not want to employ the specific skills required for a standard diagnosis and a standard treatment. It is, therefore, very important to show that, even in the affluent countries, the medical assistant can improve the health care delivery system.

Once this occurs, I hope that pressures for change will start a chain reaction which no one will be able to stop. We will then be on the right path to making this health worker a vital and efficient member of an effective care delivery system.

OPENING STATEMENT

by ABRAHAM HORWITZ, M.D.[1]

Perhaps 20 years ago a Conference on the Medical Assistant in the USA, with international participation, could not have been held. That it occurs today is evidence of the need to examine the responsibilities that the intermediate levels of health care personnel can assume in the prevention and cure of disease. The subject is of concern to both developed and developing societies in their search for immediate solutions to the most pressing health and social problems, particularly in the rural areas of the world.

It is therefore important to consider some of the reasons or circumstances that have led to this renewed interest in the intermediate as well as the auxiliary staff within the health system. The most apparent reason is the increasing imbalance in most countries between the social demand and available resources. Health is being proclaimed as a right of all— although as such it is not always clearly defined—rather than the privilege of a few. As a consequence, people are requesting equal access to the existing services, both preventive and curative. This situation has given rise to the need to plan in order to define problems and establish priorities and measurable objectives to reduce morbidity and mortality. Accordingly, health care should be perceived as a system of rational decisions with respect to both goals and investments.

In general there is no difficulty in conceiving any function, even a social one, in its totality—that is, to determine the interrelationships, the reciprocal dependence, and the effects of its various components. The health system is no exception. What is difficult is to organize and administer it for the benefit of society. The major constraint, possibly, is the rigidity of the structures—these latter being the product of the behaviour of those who direct and operate them. This applies not only to our acceptance of nonprofessional health personnel but to the assignment of their definite responsibilities as well, with or without continuous supervision. In any case they need to be part of a comprehensive approach to the solution of health problems. In other words, they should be included in the system, with their experience and their role clearly defined.

---

[1] Director, Pan American Sanitary Bureau, WHO Regional Office for the Americas, Washington, D.C.

There has been a definite change in the perception and measurement of health. Some societies are questioning the negative approach—that is to say, assessments in terms of death rates—and are considering instead whether health should not be expressed in relation to the quality of life, as a concept, as a human aspiration, and as the responsibility of each individual and the society to which he belongs. Furthermore, attempts are being made to define the quality of life and even to explore ways of measuring its components. At the same time, a definite change can be seen in the outlook of some economists regarding the productive value of the noneconomic factors of the development process, health included. When we pass from philosophical analysis to concrete programmes, the need for intermediate-level and ancillary personnel is more than apparent.

I need not elaborate on the consequences of population growth, in the face of limited resources, on the dynamics of health problems and of social wellbeing. What we should keep in mind, in discussing the role of the medical assistant and of auxiliary personnel, is that no matter how rapidly family planning programmes expand, their demographic impact will not be felt as soon as we would hope. Hence, we are forced to plan the delivery of health care services in accordance with present population trends and existing resources, particularly human ones. Once again, the health auxiliaries become indispensable.

We all welcome the vigorous movement toward community participation in the delivery of health care services that is taking shape in many countries of the world. It represents a break from paternalism, but is fraught with danger despite the opportunities it offers. We must agree with Alfred Haynes when he says, 'The consumer movement has developed in the health field as in other aspects of the social system. In the health field, it has been seen as a clear-cut reaction to medical practice which for all intents and purposes was on a course that focused less and less on people and more and more on disease.' And he adds, 'Some consider consumer involvement as a necessary evil, others have welcomed it as an educational opportunity for both the provider and the consumer. Still others have remained as neutral as possible.'[1]

It has been shown repeatedly, in urban and rural environments alike, that whenever there has been genuine motivation to increase community wellbeing, the people's response has exceeded all expectations. What is essential is to listen to them about the problems they consider most pressing and the solutions they propose, to make decisions jointly with them and to see to it that community members assume responsibility for the action to be undertaken, including the financing thereof. In sum, it has become absolutely necessary to catalyse this vast potential source of cooperation in carrying out activities for the prevention and cure of disease.

---

[1] Haynes, M. A. *Role of communities in health care.* Paper presented at the International Health Conference, sponsored by the National Council for International Health, Washington, D.C., 25–27 April, 1973, pp. 1–2.

We have interesting examples throughout the world showing how the contribution of the people increases the productivity of both professionals and nonprofessionals, thus becoming an essential component of the health care system.

Over the past 30 years, science and technology have enlarged the responsibilities of physicians and other university-trained professionals concerned with the prevention and cure of specific diseases, the organization and administration of services, and the monitoring of problems of human environment. This development has a bearing on the often asked question whether it is indispensable for physicians and other health professionals to be continuously present in order to reduce the health problems of underdeveloped countries, particularly in the rural areas. The question is far from academic. It has important implications for the education of the health professions as well as affecting the magnitude of investments in health care. If physicians were available, who could doubt their usefulness? However, the present circumstances throughout the world, and those foreseen for the next several decades, force all of us to deal with this situation through schemes far different from the orthodox ones.

As Dr Flahault has stated so well: 'The doctor's role should be reconsidered, taking into account the services that the community needs and the tasks that can be confided to other technicians. The doctor should no longer be regarded as a one-man factotum but as the leader of a team in which each member has his appropriate place.'[1]

As an example, I would like to cite the new rural health strategy that has been adopted for Latin America. It incorporates the movement toward community participation already referred to and, in addition, calls for the conversion of empirical medicine into scientific health care through the training of those who practise it. It also utilizes the health auxiliary as the focal point for both curative and preventive services provided to the people. Geography, weather, and budget permitting, the auxiliaries are supervised by nurses. Completing the scheme is a one-year to two-year rural internship for graduates in all health professions prior to their licensing. It is felt that university graduates should repay to society, through service to the poor, what society gave to them, namely, the opportunity to learn to become what they aspire to be.

The urgency of the problem in Latin America and the Caribbean area clearly stems from the situation as revealed by the following information. In 1968—we do not have any more recent figures—out of 540 297 health workers, 45% were university-trained personnel, 42% were auxiliaries, and only 12% were workers at intermediate levels. The difficulty in organizing adequate health care delivery is evident when there are not enough staff to supervise the auxiliaries and far from a minimum number of physicians to take care of even the most frequent health problems. On the other hand, it is estimated that in the Americas no fewer than 100

---

[1] Flahault, D. (1972). The case for medical assistants. *World Health*, June, pp. 8–15.

million people, equivalent to one-fifth of the total population, are without access to even a minimum health service. It is certain that other regions of the world face a comparable situation.

These are some of the factors that bear on the present situation in the health system and make it urgent to consider approaches different from the traditional ones. The purposes of this Conference on the Medical Assistant therefore take on great significance for all countries and for the World Health Organization.

With regard to the duties and training of the medical assistant, WHO has a flexible and liberal approach. Its only interest is to give the Member States, as well as all the scientists concerned with this problem, an opportunity to learn and to exchange knowledge. It is in that spirit that WHO cosponsors the present meeting and hopes that the participants will be able to adapt in their own countries, as local conditions may dictate, the ideas that emerge from the discussions here regarding the role of the medical assistant in advancing our quest for better health.

PURPOSES OF THE CONFERENCE

by *DANIEL FLAHAULT, M.D.*[1]

Both the Fogarty International Center and the World Health Organization wish to contribute to the attainment by all peoples of the highest possible level of health. This conference on the medical assistant should be placed within that broad and altruistic perspective.

First, I should like to refer to the Article 'What's in a Name' on page 1 of the June 1972 issue of *World Health*. There, the medical assistant is shown most typically as a health technician who has received eight or nine years of general education, followed by two or three years of technical training. This gives an indication of the level of the medical assistant we are discussing today, and it eliminates other levels of health aids.

The medical assistant should be able to recognize the most common diseases, to treat the simpler ones, to refer the more complicated cases to the nearest hospital or health centre, and to apply preventive measures and promote health within his area.

A large number of terms have been applied to the medical assistant as shown below:

Medical assistant	Limited physician
Medical aid	Health extension officer
Health centre superintendent	Physician assistant
Health assistant	Medex

But what we are primarily interested in is the provision of health care to the peoples of the world. Names and titles are of secondary importance. The medical assistant is one of many means to improve world health and many think that this means has not been used sufficiently. At present, only about 30 of the 137 Member states of WHO use medical assistant type personnel.

On this map of the world the black sections represent countries which at present utilize medical assistants. At the outset you can see that none of the Latin American countries train medical assistants, and not many

[1] Chief Medical Officer for Training of Auxiliary Personnel, Division of Health Manpower Development, World Health Organization, Geneva, Switzerland.

20

COUNTRIES USING MEDICAL ASSISTANTS IN 1973

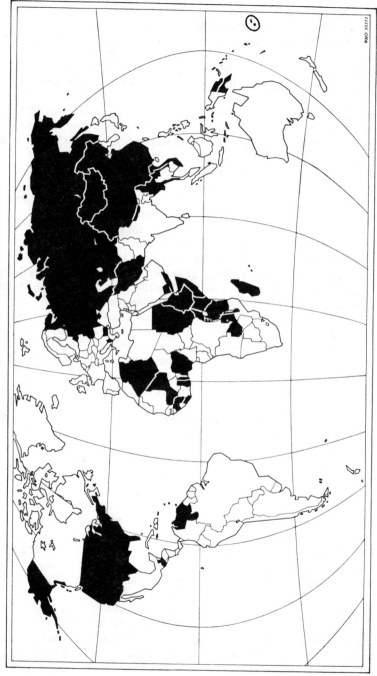

European and African countries or countries in the Pacific region or in South-East Asia either train or use medical assistants.

You can also appreciate from this map that certain countries, for example, Venezuela, train auxiliaries at a rather low level and are not shown in black for that reason. China is shown not because it trains barefoot doctors, but because, like Russia, it uses feldsher-type personnel.

Outside of those 30 countries, the tasks that medical assistants are trained to undertake are carried out by various types of personnel from the physician to the least qualified auxiliary, a solution that may be satisfactory but often is not. The quality of health services and their extension to the entire population often leaves much to be desired. The concept of the medical assistant and his place in the health team have been disputed and debated. The arguments levelled against him are not always fair and disinterested. There is no reason, on the other hand, for an indiscriminate and unreserved advocacy of the medical assistant.

We cannot be certain that the medical assistant is necessarily the best solution. But before rejecting it, it would be wise to weigh objectively and dispassionately the advantages and disadvantages. If a country wishes to use the medical assistant, his place and his role must be precisely defined as are those of any member of the health team. His training should correspond to the responsibilities and functions which have been delegated to him. His work should be guided, facilitated, assisted, supervised, and regulated. The medical assistant must not be an isolated element, nor must he be an element independent of health services. He is a cog in the wheel of health services and must be conceived of and treated as such.

If a country does not wish to use medical assistants, it should then delegate their functions to other members of the health team, and see that they are adequately trained to carry out those tasks. Only too often we still find nurses at various levels, either professional or auxiliary, who make diagnoses and prescribe treatments without having received the necessary training.

Quite recently in some schools training health personnel in Africa, European nurses of undisputed ability but lacking any training in diagnosis and therapy were teaching young African nurses their essential role and what they were to do once they were assigned to work alone in a dispensary. Their role was to diagnose and to provide treatment. Such practices, which threaten the health and life of populations, must be stopped.

In this area everything is important, particularly the training given and the role assigned to health personnel. We must try to avoid ambiguity. Some countries may find that it is prejudicial to the reputation of their health services, or an unacceptable practice, to assign to certain categories of personnel functions that have not traditionally been theirs. Thus, it is not necessarily a good practice to delegate functions of diagnosis and treatment to certain services. It is true that sometimes, owing to a lack of means or personnel, health services may be obliged to do so. But this should only be a temporary measure while a better solution is sought.

Is a nurse, whose essential functions are nursing, still a nurse once she has received supplementary training enabling her to diagnose and to provide treatment? In my opinion, she is no longer a nurse; she is something else, and a different term should be applied. Otherwise, the public may be misled.

In planning this conference, it seemed useful to bring together qualified representatives of countries who are interested in these problems and attempt to study this question, taking as a point of departure the situation existing, the experience gained, and the solutions adopted in the host country, the USA. It is true that the situation in this large country and the solutions adopted here are different from those in your countries. But our objective is not to standardize the medical assistant. It is rather to spread the idea and to show the many forms that the medical assistant can take. What is workable in the USA may not be so in other countries. But it is helpful to try to understand the reasons which have led the USA to train medical assistants and to use them under various forms with different names.

We have all been invited here to undertake a double effort of inquiry and of reflection. We hope that the results and conclusions of this conference and the conclusions that you yourselves will reach will be disseminated by you in your own countries to serve as reference points and as examples. I am deliberately avoiding the word 'model' because we are not suggesting that you copy any model for your countries. We hope that, from the information gained here, you will glean certain elements which can be transposed and adapted to your own conditions to make your own original models in accordance with the character and needs of your countries.

This conference also hopes to stimulate a two-way exchange of opinions. Our three-day programme of study will begin with several presentations designed to make you familiar with the American type of medical assistant in the context of health services and health personnel in the United States. We are counting on all of you, also, to give the conference the benefit of your experiences, difficulties, successes, failures and, in short, whatever problems you have found in your countries.

The Fogarty International Center has organized the conference in a rational way. The simultaneous interpretation system should make it possible for each one of us to express our views and to make ourselves easily understood. We are counting on you not to keep to yourself anything that you may learn from this conference but rather to use it for the benefit of your countries and, first of all, for the benefit of health services.

In inviting you to reflect on the many problems raised by medical assistants, we ask you to bear in mind three essential points.

First and foremost, we must remember that health services do not exist for the health personnel but rather for the current or potential patients and for the health of the people. We must look to the interests of the people before the interests of any particular category of health personnel.

Secondly, demographic forecasts are indispensable to those who are responsible for public health. Estimates of necessary labour for the functioning of health services serve as the basis for planning and developing the health infrastructure. As the population increases, the number of people who serve that population must increase.

TABLE 1. WORLD POPULATION PROJECTIONS (LOWER ESTIMATE)

Year	Total world population (millions)	World rural population[1] (millions)	Rural population as % of total population
1970	3572.5	2545.4	71
1980	4231.9	2847.3	67
1990	4938.0	3123.2	63
2000	5670.4	3378.1	59

Source: United Nations Population Division (1969) Unpublished document.
[1] Including rural populations living in communities of less than 20 000.

Table 1 shows that, in 1970, the total population of the world was about 3572 million inhabitants. of which 71%, that is 2500 million, lived in rural areas. According to a conservative estimate by the USA itself, the total population will reach 5670 million in the year 2000.

A maximum estimate would be that the world population will exceed 7000 million inhabitants by the year 2000. This means that to achieve the present level and quality of service, health personnel must increase by 60% in the case of the conservative estimate, and by more than 100% if the maximum estimate proves to be correct.

TABLE 2. WORLD RURAL POPULATION PROJECTIONS (LOWER ESTIMATE)

Year	World rural population (1)	In more developed regions (2)	In less developed regions[1] (3)	(3) as % of (1)
1970	2545.4	538.8	2006.6	79
1980	2847.3	545.7	2401.6	81
1990	3123.2	548.6	2574.6	82
2000	3378.1	550.1	2828.0	84

Source: United Nations Population Division (1969) Unpublished document.
[1] Africa, Asia (excluding Japan), Central America, South America (excluding temperate zone), Oceania (excluding Australia and New Zealand).

Table 2 shows that while the rural population of the developed countries will not grow appreciably, the rural population of the less developed regions will increase by nearly 50%. If we do not wish to be content with simply maintaining health services in their present state and wish to improve these health services, we must envisage an increase in personnel. Medical assistants have a role to play in these projected increases. It is an important and, perhaps, vital role, particularly in certain areas.

Population growth in the world between the years 1960 and 1968 was analysed in the *Fourth Report on the World Health Situation* 1960–1968[1] in order to determine its effect on health services as well as on morbidity and social conditions. This study showed that it is only in the most advanced countries that the development of health services keeps in step with population growth. In most of the developing countries, it will be very difficult for the increase in the numbers of nurses, dentists and doctors to follow the population growth. Extension of services can come only from a multiplication of the possibilities of professional training and from the utilization of auxiliaries.

My third and final point concerns the central role which medical assistants can play in development by virtue of their assignment in the front line of health services, their responsibilities for promoting health, and their privileged position in the community. The medical assistant may be an instrument of development of health services in either rural or urban areas. In the rural areas he may head a team in charge of a dispensary, while in urban areas he may serve as assistant to the physician whom he relieves of routine tasks, thus allowing him to devote his time to work which requires his particular competence. In both cases the medical assistant increases the effectiveness of health services and may promote their qualitative and quantitative development.

In addition, the medical assistant can and must be used as an element of community development. The medical assistant in the community often becomes a prominent person who is respected and listened to because of his better than average education and his effective techniques. He knows the people, he listens to them, and he understands them better than anyone else. He is, therefore, in a favourable position to influence and motivate them, to stimulate them, and to channel the ideas and concerns of the community.

To learn about the solutions adopted in other countries, to share with others the experience gained in your own country, to reflect together on problems which affect all of us, to recognize that there is no ideal or universal solution, to assess the advantages and disadvantages of medical assistants, and to bear in mind certain basic concerns—these are the objectives and the *raisons d'être* of this conference. We hope that, in pursuing them, we shall help to extend the possible role of medical assistants in the improvement of health services.

---

[1] *Off. Rec. Wld Hlth Org.*, 1971, No. 192.

HEALTH SERVICES IN THE USA: TRENDS IN THE EDUCATION AND TRAINING OF HEALTH PERSONNEL

by LEONARD D. FENNINGER, M.D.[1]

First, may I stress the point that the individual members of each society are responsible for their own health, for the development of health services, and for the provision of resources for the care of the sick and the prevention of illness.

Second, it is important to recognize that all health care really stems from the culture in which it is given. Therefore, cultural variations are reflected in what each nation or group does in providing care and in accepting standards of care.

Third, there is a long history among all peoples of the use of different kinds of persons with different kinds of training to assist in providing health services and in preventing illness. We may tend to forget that there were probably physician's assistants at the time of Cro-Magnon man 25 000 years ago when the Cro-Magnon shaman priest had a small boy who carried his bag of necessary instruments for his practice of healing as then conceived.

So there is really nothing new about having different kinds of people, with different backgrounds and different training, share in the provision of health care. Each of us has something to learn from others and also something to learn from past experience, an exercise that human beings seem to find particularly difficult.

Health services in any given nation are greatly modified by the culture and the views of people living within a particular region and organized in a particular way. It may therefore be of interest to outline briefly some of my views on how the USA arrived at its present position with respect to the use of various middle-level medical personnel. It should also be pointed out that the problems of health care in the United States are qualitatively, although not quantitatively, similar to those in other countries. The same kinds of questions are raised: Is care available to a person when it is needed? Is the quality of care satisfactory? Can the cost of care be properly borne by the society whose members are to receive it?

[1] Director of Graduate Medical Education, American Medical Association, Chicago, Ill.

The USA is quite different, of course, from other nations in its origins and in organization. The present arrangements for health care stem from colonial times before the United States of America existed. We began as a colony of England, and there were very few people trained in any professional field at the time the country was settled.

Therefore, the various arrangements and accommodations made in order that society could function at all were quite different from what many of us would now consider suitable health care. From the beginning, there have been debates about the degree of responsibility for the provision of health care, and particularly medical care, which should rest with the general public and the community and the degree of responsibility which should rest with the individual or his family, or with private enterprise, that is, business, industry, and private institutions. That debate still goes on; it is by no means resolved.

There has been a gradual evolution in the preparation of health personnel in the USA. Because of the very small number of well prepared professional people in the colonies and because, in our early history, energies were devoted, particularly in New England, to surviving in a rather hostile land, most of the training of health personnel took the form of apprenticeships. In the 17th and 18th centuries, a very small number of people from the colonies went to Europe for their training.

It is a relatively recent development in the USA to have within the educational system training programmes for all levels of health personnel. But this issue has by no means been finally settled in the USA, since a great number of people who serve as providers of medical and health care, particularly in hospitals, are trained on an apprenticeship basis even today. Nevertheless, there have been increasing links between educational institutions, the health occupations and professions, and the agencies which deliver health care. These groups have joined together to provide sound training for the people who are going to participate in health services at every level, whether as direct practitioners or in community health, sanitation, preventive medicine, administration, finance, or organization. We have moved more and more, particularly in the last 50 years, towards an educational system that prepares people for their practical or clinical experience in a health service institution linked to the educational institution.

It is important to bear this relationship in mind, particularly in discussing some of the programmes that are now under way to prepare middle-level medical personnel in this country.

Since our early history, there has been considerable debate regarding standards and who should be responsible for establishing them. In many nations, the standards of performance are established by the national government. But in the USA, this responsibility has been largely left in nongovernmental hands. The standards for physicians, for example, have been established by organizations of physicians and medical educators. The same may be said for standards of performance of dentists and of nurses.

In a sense, the federal and state governments recognize these standards through the health professions practice acts of the states, which then determine who is eligible and who is not eligible to perform certain duties within the state. Nonetheless, the establishment of fundamental standards and much of the control of standard setting have remained with the professions. This circumstance has created both benefits and problems, as is almost always the case with any standard setting.

Education has also been a function of the states and the private sector rather than the national government in the USA. Much of the education, both historically and at the present time, is provided in institutions that are supported from nongovernmental sources.

We have a very mixed educational system. The contribution from professional groups is primarily in the setting of standards for the health professions and occupations. The codification of performance and minimum requirements for practitioners is set by the states. In fact, it is only since 1965, when the 'Medicare' legislation was passed, that the Federal Government has had any means of directly influencing the standards of performance of practitioners in the USA. Only when the Federal Government actually became involved in payment for services did it set a series of standards of performance which could be generally applicable throughout all states; in fact, these standards are applicable only to services to people eligible for support under Federal programmes.

Once this was done, the standard of performance began to influence all other standards of performance. But in the strict sense, the Federal standards apply only in the case of beneficiaries of payments by the Federal Government and do not apply to services given to people who are insured by private insurance systems, or by workmen's compensation, or by the multitude of other arrangements we have for payment of care in this country.

Our system of government, like any other system of government, profoundly affects the ways in which care is given. Because we hope somehow that promises made during an election campaign can become fact through a particular administration's initiatives, we have tended to raise disproportionately the expectations and the demand for more and better care. As a nation and as a people, we have tended not to make the investments necessary for the fulfilment of these promises.

In the development of the Constitution, through which the Government of the USA was created, much of the individual independence of the colonies was preserved, particularly in matters of education; education became essentially a responsibility of the states and not of the Federal Government. The Federal Government has recently become more involved in the support of education, but it has done so while maintaining the assumption that the basic educational responsibilities lie with each of the states of the USA rather than with the national government.

At the same time, influenced by traditions from England, we have long had a strong private, philanthropic contribution to health services and to education for health services. We are at present in a transitional period; this is one of the reasons for our being uncomfortable in dealing with some health issues. We still tend to think that the provision of health services, and particularly the provision of medical and hospital care, is essentially a charitable act. We feel this emotionally, whereas we know in our minds that this is not the case. The conflict between heart and head is often one of the most painful conflicts in trying to come to some kind of social decision.

Let me say a word or two about the organization of health services in the USA before I close with a general discussion of the education and training of various kinds of health personnel. Among the current issues that are being debated in governmental bodies such as our Congress, in state assemblies and legislatures, in educational institutions, and in health service institutions, as well as by industrialists, businessmen, and the public is, first of all, that of the availability of health services and particularly the availability of physicians and medical services. This issue is uppermost in people's minds. People tend to think in terms of episodes of illness rather than in terms of continuity of health.

Second is the matter of the quality and quantity of services available to all segments of the population. Can one, in fact, distribute health services of good quality to everybody in a given nation, or will we continue to have the degrees of unevenness which we have had in the past? Again, cultural aspects enter very strongly into this question because, in our case, health is given very great importance, particularly by planners, the better educated, and the economically more comfortable people. (The priorities are different in other groups.) The question of quality and quantity of services and their equitable distribution is thus second in our consideration.

Third is the question of costs and the means of meeting them, which I perceive as a worldwide concern. It is a concern of increasing moment as the demand for medical and health services rises and as the organization of services becomes more complex. So we share with the rest of the world these common concerns. Perhaps the emphasis we place on them is somewhat different from that of other nations, but these are common themes throughout the entire world.

Health services are organized in many different ways in the USA, simply because they have sprung from many different social backgrounds and different kinds of geographical and economic settings with different demands.

The whole concept of medicine has changed remarkably as we have become more industrialized and as medical and scientific research has given us knowledge and tools that we simply did not possess before.

In general, public and community health services in the USA are functions of local government, state government and, to a lesser extent, of the Federal Government. They are concerned on the one hand with the quality of the environment—prevention of air and water pollution, evacuation of solid wastes, sanitation, safety of food and drugs, and control of toxic substances—and, on the other hand, with the prevention of illness among communities and populations.

Family and personal health have been organized in a somewhat different fashion. We see, for example, the hospital playing a greater role as a base for giving care, but we see at the same time a public demand for more and more care to be given outside the hospital, despite the fact that the public has strongly supported hospital development. The hospital's role has increased inevitably with the growth in medical knowledge and technology and in the number of different skills that have to be brought to bear on an individual problem. Only an organization such as the hospital could bring together the resources necessary to attack complex problems.

In the USA we have tended also to use the hospital to attack simple problems which might well have been cared for in another setting if our insurance mechanisms had evolved to pay for ambulatory, out-of-hospital care. But again, more or less by historical accident, most of the medical insurance and hospital insurance policies and concepts arose during the depression of the early 1930s. They were not conceived as a means for insuring or maintaining health but as a means for offsetting the economic disaster of illness. What we call health insurance in the USA really started as illness insurance, with a hospital emphasis that has persisted to this day.

Therefore, the importance of the hospital has increased not only for sound professional and scientific reasons; its importance has also been emphasized by the methods of payment for medical services. The demand for continuity of care and prevention of illness requires, of course, organization of care that is *not* hospital-based. Hospitals are at present geared to deal with episodes of illness and, in the USA, they are particularly geared to the most serious medical problems. They are not designed for day-to-day, long-term relationships with an individual or with his family. Hospitals have, of course, been the sites of creation of what some people choose to call 'health teams' because it is comparatively easy to organize groups of people from different disciplines in the setting of the hospital. There is an increasing demand for, and an increasing attempt at present to create, 'health teams' outside hospitals—in physicians' offices, in neighbourhood health clinics or in group practices—a trend which influences the education and training of middle-level personnel.

There are also trends toward group practice in which multi-specialty groups of physicians come together and contract to provide medical care on a prepaid basis with defined costs for specified services for the period of the agreement—this is in contrast to our Blue Cross plans for hospital insurance which insure for cost without having any control over what the cost is. The prepaid group plans control cost by determining what services will be given at what level of payment and then commit themselves through contract to provide that service at that level.

The most serious problems in medical care, as I have said, have to do with distribution and availability of medical services. This is a reflection of the distribution and availability of competent personnel.

We have shortages of three different kinds. We have shortages by geographical location, most marked, of course, in the low-income rural areas and the seriously low-income areas of our cities which, in the past 20 years, have received a major migration of people from rural areas, mostly people of low economic background. The problems of the cities and the delivery of care are related to a profound cultural change. Many people in the USA fail to realize that the migration from rural to urban areas and the migration of the poor to the cities constitute the largest single migration that has ever occurred in our history. We tend to forget that this contributes considerably to our present social and health problems.

In addition to shortages of services linked to geographical location and economic status, there are also shortages of the services of different specialists. Many communities have more than enough physicians to meet needs in certain medical specialties; other communities are totally lacking in these special services. Much of the current debate concerns the means not only to readjust the geographical and economic distribution of health personnel but also to modify the choice of specialty of the particular health professional so that his or her special ability fits with the needs of people rather than with his or her particular interest. This is an inordinately difficult problem.

There is also the point of how effectively services are used. The question is not only whether a particular service is needed, but whether responsibilities are suitably delegated to people who can assume them effectively, and whether care given by one group is in any way coordinated with care given by another.

Another very important question is whether people who make use of these services really know what the services are and how to make effective use of them. We tend to forget that most of the fundamental decisions with respect to the use of health services are made by nonprofessional people. These decisions are made by citizens; they are made by members of communities. As professionals, we tend to think we make the decisions. In fact, the public makes them. The better informed the public is, the wiser those decisions will be. There is the problem of broadening the understanding and knowledge about health services of the people who need and demand them.

In attempting to deal with some of the distribution problems and the availability of timely medical care, people in the health professions are changing roles at a relatively rapid rate. The functions of nurses, for example, have expanded tremendously in the last 20 years in many communities, although in rural areas in the USA nurses have long dealt with family and community health to a greater extent than have physicians. Nurses' roles are also changing within the organization of administration of health services in general.

The physician's assistant and other middle-level people who are educated and trained to assume, in a responsible and competent fashion, functions formerly performed by other professional groups will be discussed at greater length, together with the question of specialization and of the organization of health personnel and health services into groups. We also have an increasing number of technical specialists working in organized settings; they will be alluded to but their functions will not be discussed in detail. Certain specialized functions connected with the administrative legal and social aspects of health care are becoming much more important, and special training is now required and is being given for them.

As a nation and as individuals, we are debating various plans for payment for services. Currently, there are plans in which individuals or families pay for their care. There are also plans in which employers pay for a portion of care. There are plans in which unions pay for a portion of health care from dues paid by their members. Insurance is provided by private insurance companies. The social security insurance system of Medicare is operated and directed by the Federal Government. Joint sharing of expense and cost between the Federal Government and the states for certain eligible populations occurs through Medicaid. And there is direct provision of health care by Federal and state governments for beneficiaries defined by the Federal or state laws.

Finally, let me say something about the education and training of health professionals in the USA. Since much of the education and training of people other than physicians is related inevitably to the training of physicians, who in the USA bear the final responsibility for medical care, I would like to say a few words about medical education and training and also about nursing education and training and the training of intermediate health personnel.

Medical education in the USA is a fusion of the university-based education of middle Europe with the hospital-based, more or less apprentice system that was in effect in the British Isles in the late nineteenth century and with our frontier medicine. Frontier medicine was the medicine of expediency, a phenomenon of our early history that was due to the expansion and settlement of large, relatively sparsely populated parts of the country.

It was not until 1920 that an effort was made to link medical education to university education as a general pattern in the USA. This followed by a decade the report that Mr Abraham Flexner made for the Carnegie Commission on Higher Education regarding medical education in the USA.

The linkage that occurred with universities in the education of the physician was initially a linkage of two relatively independent bodies. But more and more attempts are being made to unify the whole of medical education from entrance to college to the conclusion of postdoctoral training, and to link the institutions in which this training occurs to give some rational continuity as regards both experience and increasing responsibility in the course of medical and health studies.

The Federal Government is now indirectly fostering such links by providing funds to the institutions making them.

Changes are taking place in the medical school curriculum itself. There is a strong push now to shorten the period of formal medical education in the USA. My own view is that the length of an educational period is largely a function of the culture and the economy of the nation. A nation that can afford to have large segments of its population not engaged in immediate production for a fairly long time tends to prolong the formal educational period. A nation that does not have such human or material resources tends to shorten the educational period. But we are making a conscious effort to reduce the period of formal education, partly because of public pressures to increase the number of health personnel and partly because some medical educators think that the time of medical students has not been used as effectively as it might.

A second trend is to give medical students more extensive experience of ambulatory health care. This is occurring to some extent through revision of the functions or changes in the attitudes of clinical services and emergency departments in the hospitals where our medical students have traditionally been trained.

Physicians in the community are participating in the education of the medical student, with the student working either in the physician's office, in group practice, or in neighbourhood health centres operated by the community in conjunction with educational and patient-care institutions. These are examples of attempts to give medical students an experience in continuity of care and in the care of patients who are upright rather than lying in bed.

There is also a trend to increase the amount of elective time for the student so that he himself may choose what he wishes to study for at least part of his education and may express his own abilities and inclinations during his time in medical school.

A significant trend at the moment is the attempt to educate the physician together with other types of health personnel so that he will work more effectively with them in the provision of good health care.

Parallel to these changes in the medical curriculum are a number of modifications of internship and residency programmes. Medical schools are assuming more responsibility for this post-medical-school period of training than they did in the past when hospital and professional groups had almost sole responsibility for the postgraduate training of physicians in the USA.

There is also a good deal of discussion about other types of institutions and agencies that might participate in the postdoctoral clinical training of physicians. There is, at the moment, a strong movement to develop programmes of family practice. Special Federal legislation and financial support exist to encourage family practice education in medical schools and hospitals, and in health institutions, organizations, and agencies in the community.

Recently, both state and Federal governments have given increasing support to medical education in the United States. As far as the Federal

Government is concerned, this development dates back less than 15 years. The individual states, on the other hand, have been major supporters of medical education for a much longer time.

The proportion of private support for medical education is declining compared to the funds from state governments and the Federal Government, although the total dollar amount of private funding has increased. As the funds from the Federal Government rise, the latter's influence on medical education is obviously apt to rise as well. I think we will see some periods of rather difficult adjustment, since Federal purposes and those of medical schools are not always entirely consonant.

Nursing education, which was originally an apprentice system in the hospital, has come more and more to be based in educational institutions in the form of two-year or four-year college programmes. A declining number of students elect to enter three-year hospital training programmes, rather than a college or a university.

The number of students entering two-year and four-year nursing programmes is increasing rapidly, partly because of the changes in nursing and partly because our young people choose to go to college rather than enter an apprentice type of training,

The functions of nursing are changing quite rapidly and, therefore, some substantial educational and curricular modifications are occurring in both the two-year and the four-year programmes.

Increasingly, nurses are entering specialized practice reflecting the specialized practice of medicine that has developed in the USA. The role of the public health nurse is increasing rather than diminishing as she becomes the health counsellor for the people who need her services in a community where, frequently, a physician is lacking.

Nurses have assumed major responsibility for long-term care, ambutory care, and continuity of care; this calls for substantial reorganization of nursing service administration in virtually all of our institutions.

We are examining the function of nursing services in our primary and secondary schools and in industry. These are fields where a large number of nurses serve but have provided less community service and continuity of health care than, I believe, they are capable of providing.

Specialized technicians, or other more generally prepared people who are participating in health care, are also being trained increasingly in educational institutions; their clinical experience is being provided in an organization or hospital affiliated with the educational institution and linked with the educational programme. Many of these training and educational programmes are, at the moment, rather experimental and vary considerably not only within the USA but even within individual states. A number of different paths are being followed, and different educational patterns and content and different settings for education are being tried out.

One important consideration in the training and use of middle-level personnel is the degree of organization of the setting in which they will function. The more organized the setting, the more likely they are to have specialized functions and to have other skilled people to support them, to give advice and counsel, and to participate in care.

The type of education and the type of experience of the middle-level person have to be developed in view of the setting in which the person's skills will be used and the functions actually performed.

The functions to be performed, for example, in rural New Mexico would be quite different from those in Bethesda, Maryland. This has to be taken into account in education. How will a person develop good judgement and acquire enough information to respond to the medical needs of the public? How can he be given the kind of experience that will allow him to work well in a setting quite different from that in which he received his training?

We are debating the degree of capability of so-called middle-level health workers, the means to test their competence and ability, and how to determine what levels of responsibility they are capable of accepting. We are trying to work out the degree to which the public will accept such people in lieu of a physician, even one to whom the public is accustomed in name but may never see in fact. We are particularly concerned about the problem of the physicians who are going to have to work with such people. Physicians are notoriously not very flexible in sharing responsibility with others. The very nature of their profession tends to make them into the kind of person who discharges responsibility well but finds it difficult to share it.

Because of all the changes that are occurring in the absence of a series of generally accepted standards, payment mechanisms, types of services or eligibility for them, we have not settled the question of quality. Who will determine quality? What are the criteria for quality? Who will be permitted to perform various functions of medical care? How much of the functions of the various health personnel will be governmentally and how much will be professionally determined? To what degree will the public have a direct voice in setting standards of practice and in excluding from practice people whom the public deems to be inadequate?

DEFINITION OF TERMS

by *DOUGLAS FENDERSON*, *Ph.D.*[1]

Dr Flahault has illustrated the large number of names used for medical assistants throughout the world and has recommended the adoption of a definition for the purposes of this meeting. A confusing array of names and titles has been applied in this country to a large and variable class of clinical-medical workers whose level of preparation and responsibility is similar to that in Dr Flahault's definition but is less than that of the fully licensed medical practitioner.

This family of middle-level clinical workers, as described in the Rosinski–Spencer study[2] 'seem to perform at a similar medical level. No uniform title may justly identify these personnel. Many perform at the level of the medical doctor/general practitioner, while others are specialists.'

To simplify their presentation, Rosinski and Spencer used a single descriptive label—the assistant medical officer. Fendall, in his recent multinational report[3] and discussion, uses the term 'medical auxiliary,' a term which covers a range of clinical and technical roles. He uses this term to imply 'a clear and wide gap between the auxiliary on the one hand, and the professional or paraprofessional on the other.'

Fendall believes that terminology in this area is extremely important if misunderstandings are to be avoided, and he illustrates this with the term 'medical assistant.' He notes that its meaning may range from a receptionist–helper in a physician's office to a substitute for the physician as used in East Africa.

Even though Fendall considers auxiliaries to be separated by a clear and wide gap from even the paraprofessional level, he notes in his recent book that in the countries he studied, 'possibly 5 to 10% of the patients need more knowledgeable attention than can be given by the auxiliary.'

Fendall recommends the use of more descriptive names in particular settings for various types of clinical workers. And indeed there is no shortage of these, as has been illustrated earlier here.

---

[1] Bureau of Health Manpower Education, National Institutes of Health, Bethesda, Md.
[2] Rosinski, E. F., & Spencer, F. J. (1967) The training and duties of the medical auxiliary known as the assistant medical officer. *Amer. J. publ. Hlth*, 57, 1663–1669.
[3] Fendall, N. R. E. (1972) *Auxiliaries in health care; programs in developing countries*, Baltimore & London, Johns Hopkins Press (Josiah Macy Foundation).

Programmes supported by the Bureau of Health Manpower Education[1] of the National Institutes of Health include a total of 33 different descriptive names or titles—8 for non-nursing physician's assistants, 19 for variations on the nursing theme, and 6 within the field of middle-level dental auxiliaries.

Part of this problem of names and labels results from differences in systems and in availability of higher education, and part from the strong trend in some of the more developed countries towards academic programmes that overtrain persons for relatively straightforward vocational and technical tasks. Nor is this true in the health professions alone.

The purpose of this brief statement is not to suggest a new name or title. One of the participants in this meeting, Dr Henry Silver, has suggested a descriptive label, 'syniatrist.' I will not emphasize any particular name, but I would like to characterize this role as it has been developing in this country.

Most of our programmes, at least those for which Federal support has been available, have emphasized primary, ambulatory medical care. They are largely directed toward the so-called low-access or underserved areas of our country and were seen initially as a countervailing force to over-specialization in medicine and to geographic maldistribution.

The role, as it has emerged in the USA, generally includes the following abilities:

To take a general medical history and perform a physical examination.
To order, and in some instances perform, frequently required laboratory tests and procedures.
To organize findings in an accurate and logical manner for review by the physician.
To provide preventive care and treatment for a defined range of conditions or problems, such as treatment under standing orders.
To apply therapeutic measures as directed by the physician.
To identify patients requiring more precise medical evaluation or treatment.
To monitor the progress of patients, particularly those having stable chronic conditions.
To keep accurate and appropriate records of services performed.

Dr Flahault made the point that, if one looks around the world, one finds a large number of such workers, labelled and defined in rather special ways. Some of their titles are given in the following list.

Professional	Primex (USA)
Feldsher (USSR)	Ancillary
Near doctor (South Africa)	Medex (USA)
Sub-professional	Assistant medical officer (Fiji)
Barefoot doctor (China)	Medical aid (India)

---

[1] Now Bureau of Health Resources Development of Health Resources Administration.

Médecin africain (French-
    speaking African countries)   Nurse practitioner
Health assistant   Physician's assistant
Paramedic   Junior auxiliary
Allied health worker   Middle auxiliary
Health extension worker   Senior auxiliary
Medical assistant   Limited physician
          Auxiliary worker

Nurse practitioners have been assuming greater responsibility in the provision of primary ambulatory medical care to supplement the nursing services typically and traditionally associated with the profession. If one matches any name in the column on the left below with the word 'nurse', plus any name from the column on the right below, one may generate 55 possible combinations of nurse practitioner.

Family
Paediatric
Geriatric
Primary care
Community health   specialist
Ambulatory   nurse   practitioner
Docent   associate
Comprehensive   supervisor
School   clinician
Rural
Clinical

There are, in addition, names such as primary health practitioner, family health specialist (worker), nurse-physician's assistant, nurse-midwife, and obstetrical nurse practitioner.

The more common names for workers in this country whose background has generally not included nursing are derived from a combination of any label in the column on the left below with any label in the column on the right below, except that one title, 'Medex', stands alone.

Physician's
Physicians'
Community health   assistant
Family health   associate
Clinical   medic
Medical services

In dentistry, several terms are derived by combining extended (or expanded) duty (or function) with:

auxiliary
assistant
hygienist
therapist

and in addition there are titles such as:

> dental therapist
> dental nurse
> periodontal therapist
> paedodontal therapist

Professor Timothy Baker has pointed out that many of the developing countries use technicians with less training in providing medical care than has been defined for this particular meeting. Dr Flahault's clarification with regard to the Latin American countries is instructive on that point. I think it is abundantly clear to those of you who have travelled a lot and have studied the available literature that in some instances—and I quote Dr Fendall again—'The least well-prepared get the shortest training and the lowest pay for the most difficult of the jobs.'

DISCUSSION

Chairman: RAMON VILLARREAL, M.D.[1]

VILLARREAL: The conference is open for discussion, comments, or questions concerning the previous speakers' remarks.

BEAUSOLEIL (*Ghana*): In view of the availability of health facilities and resources and the state of development of the health services, there does not appear to be an urgent need for the development of a cadre of intermediate-level health workers. If the aim is to correct imbalance between the different socio-economic classes and different geographical regions, then one can visualize the adoption of other approaches for the solution of the problem. It would be interesting to know what efforts have been made to correct maldistribution of health services.

One approach might be the introduction of legislation to prevent new persons from setting up practice in areas which are adequately provided for.

FENNINGER (*USA*): There are efforts to attract health personnel into areas of scarce medical services by altering the distribution of payments for services. There have also been discussions of differential payments according to specialty.

Because of the system of government and the private-citizen–public-responsibility relationships in the USA, and because a practitioner who cares for a patient outside the hospital also cares for that patient in the hospital, it is very difficult for the Federal Government or a state government to interfere directly in the distribution of physicians either by specialty or by geographical location. This is socially and politically unacceptable at the moment.

We are currently seeking ways that are acceptable to the public and to the professions to change methods of payment, to change the community resources to attract health personnel, and to persuade the medical specialty groups and the hospitals to modify their requirements for training, to modify the ways in which training is given, and to encourage people to go into the scarcer specialties and avoid specialties where there is an abundance of personnel.

But the Federal Government does not run any health service except for the Armed Forces, American Indians, and certain other groups that are specified by law as being beneficiaries of Federal programmes. In this respect the USA is quite different from many other nations. There is no national health service in the country.

It was in 1971, I think, that Congress passed a law for a national health service on an emergency basis. This law is being administered by the Health Services and Mental Health Administration[2] of the Department of Health, Education,

---

[1] Pan American Health Organization, Washington, D.C.
[2] Now the Alcohol, Drug Abuse, and Mental Health Administration.

and Welfare. The statute provides that members of the United States Public Health Service may be assigned to areas of scarce medical services and give care with the expectation that some persons assigned to such areas will remain there.

At the moment this is a very small and essentially experimental programme. Really it is testing the social and political climate to determine the degree of acceptability of this kind of Federal intervention in what has been a highly independent, highly individual choice by the physician of both his specialty and the location of his practice.

ACUÑA (*Mexico*): I would like to clarify two points. I understood Dr Flahault to say that in Latin America there is no need at the present time for medical assistants. This is certainly not so. Apart from Venezuela, which Dr Flahault mentioned, I can refer to El Salvador, for instance, which in 1954 instituted a programme of medical assistants or nursing aids in the WHO health demonstration area. Brazil has similar programmes in collaboration with the Agency for International Development and other institutions. In Peru and Colombia programmes of this kind were instituted years ago. In my own country, Mexico, for a long time nurse's aids, male and female, have been trained to undertake certain activities in rural areas and sometimes in urban areas; they work under the close supervision of a physician. It should be emphasized, however, that these are not generalized programmes on a national basis but simply at the district level.

The other point I wish to clarify is Dr Fenninger's statement that the higher the level of national economy, the shorter the period of training of medical personnel. May I ask if my interpretation is correct or is it *vice versa*?

FENNINGER (*USA*): I intended to say the reverse. Countries with the largest surplus in their economies can and do afford a longer period of education for a larger group of people in the health field than those with more limited economies.

FLAHAULT (*WHO, Geneva*): I am grateful to Dr Acuña for giving me an opportunity to clarify a point related to the objectives of this conference. I did not say that there was no need for medical assistants in Latin America. I simply regretted the fact that, on the map presented, with the exception of Guatemala, there were no Latin American countries with medical assistant programmes as defined by the World Health Organization, that is a medical assistant of a high level. It is not the same as in Venezuela where the training of medical aids is a six-month programme, whereas the training of medical assistants requires two or three years and sometimes even more, with a general basic education of eight or nine years.

We must not confuse the basic level medical aid, like the barefoot doctor in China and similar examples in many other countries, with the high-level medical assistant.

This conference is centred on the high-level medical assistant, the one that we call the intermediate level of health personnel as indicated in the title and described in the June 1972 issue of *World Health*.

NATHANIELS (*Togo*): In Togo for the first time, we have just begun an experiment with what we call medical assistants. Earlier in the discussion, it was said that some are in favour of this intermediate-level type of personnel while others oppose it. But consider what Dr Flahault said a moment ago—that about 71 % of the world's population lives in rural areas. As far as Togo is concerned, it is not possible to provide the rural population with qualified physicians, hence the necessity to train well-qualified medical assistants who can give adequate health care. More than once a week, on the average, we see acute cases in which the diagnosis and treatment were incorrect, with the result that surgical intervention becomes necessary. If we had well-trained and qualified people, that sort of difficulty could be avoided. Diagnosis could be made by qualified people who could refer patients to proper health centres.

SOOPIKIAN (*Iran*): When Dr Fenninger was speaking of the new trends in the USA, he described the training of medical assistants and mentioned how effectively the medical manpower was used. In order that the physician may be freed for more specialized and higher tasks, he has been relieved of those that can be performed by a middle-level assistant. In developing this programme, was an analysis made of the task performed by the physician? Is this just a short-term plan because of the shortage of doctors? Or is this a new category of health worker that will continue in the health system permanently?

FENNINGER (*USA*): I wish that one could say that the programmes had come into being after some kind of logical analysis of the functions of physicians and other health personnel, and that the training programmes had been designed to fill in the gaps or to enable personnel to assume functions and responsibilities that could be transferred from one health professional to another. In fact, many of the programmes were a response to public pressure for more medical services and were conceived, and actually fostered by certain branches of the Federal Government, as a short-term measure to help meet an immediate problem.

That is not true of all programmes. Some were based on a careful examination of the current functions of various health personnel, particularly physicians and nurses, and were designed to supplement and complement those functions by training a person to assume certain specific responsibilities.

PRINCIPAL TRAINING PROGRAMMES IN THE USA

PHYSICIAN'S ASSISTANT—PHYSICIAN'S ASSOCIATE

by E. HARVEY ESTES, Jr, M.D.[1]

I would like to introduce this group to one broad type of intermediate-level health worker, the physician's assistant, a relatively new addition to the medical scene in the USA.

My task is considerably complicated by the realization that many of you have had experience with intermediate-level health workers, assistant medical officers, and other similar categories, long before the concept was established here. Moreover, many of you come from areas in which the organization of care and the roles of the various professionals within that organization are quite different from what they are in the USA.

Dr Fenninger has properly stated that medical care is a product of the culture that supports it. This is pertinent in considering the development of the physician's assistant in this country.

As a nation, we have a tradition of using our resources in a lavish and wasteful way. Our national philosophy with regard to health has been true to this tradition. As a nation, we tend to consider the best medical care as that which is delivered by a highly trained specialist in a highly differentiated institution, such as a hospital.

In medicine, as in most other areas, there is a quality–quantity trade-off. In the USA the choice has always been strongly on the side of quality, that is, a higher order of training, more sophisticated technical equipment, a more structured type of system, and so forth.

It is only relatively recently that we have come to realize the extent of the gap between the services and those needed, particularly in rural areas and inner city areas, and have been willing to look at some of the alternatives that might exist.

Medical manpower, like money and gasoline, is a resource which has practical, finite limits, and which should be conserved. As we have learned this, we have also realized that many tasks that have been traditionally performed by the doctor can be done equally well, or perhaps even better, by those with considerably less training.

This is perhaps the real significance of the programmes that we are discussing today. They have emerged as a result of a realization that the

---

[1] Duke University Medical Center, Durham, North Carolina.

demand for health services is unlimited while the supply of medical manpower does have limits, or at least the economic means for generating and supporting that manpower has limits. As a result, we are now able to consider some of the alternatives.

It was this realization that led to the first physician's assistant training programme in the USA. In 1966, Dr Eugene Stead, who was then the Chairman of the Department of Medicine at Duke University, became acutely aware of the tremendous burden faced by the general physicians in our largely rural area of the USA. The output of highly trained specialists and subspecialists by all the medical schools in that area had been absorbed into the larger cities, leaving the rural areas of North Carolina with a severe shortage of medical services. This is a specific example of the geographical maldistribution of physicians that has been mentioned before.

It was also realized that no generally trained assistant was available to the doctor. A variety of specially trained laboratory technicians, radiological technicians, and so forth were able to assist with their very specific services. There were also nurses, almost all with exclusively hospital training. Moreover, the shortage of nursing manpower in our area limited the availability of nursing services even within the hospitals.

For these reasons, Dr Stead proposed that Duke University begin to train a general assistant for the doctor, capable of performing many of the tasks that were then considered the province of the doctor himself and able to function in any of the settings in which the doctor operates.

In the USA, the doctor moves readily from his office and the patient's home into the hospital and back again. He is not confined to one geographical location. One of Dr Stead's objectives, then, was to train an assistant who could move readily with the doctor from one of these settings to another.

Accordingly, in 1966, the Duke physician's assistant programme, or 'PA' programme, was born. Because of the previously-mentioned shortage of nurses and because of the desire for maximum geographical and temporal flexibility, it was decided that men from backgrounds as military hospital corpsmen would be recruited into the programme. They became its substrate, if you will. The first class was quite small, three in number.

I emphasize that the programme began without those studies which were cited in an earlier discussion as being highly desirable. There was no formal exploration of the need, the acceptance, the type of task delegation, and so forth. There was also no extensive study of the curriculum and how it might meet these needs.

The curriculum was constructed in the beginning by experienced medical educators after consultation with practising physicians in the area, it being understood that the process and the product could and would change as we learned more about the need and the fit between this need, the educational programme, and the products of the programme.

The faculty in this original programme was the medical faculty, and the teaching techniques were those which had become established within the medical school. The curriculum required two years. There were nine months of didactic lectures and fifteen months of practical work in caring for patients in various medical settings.

The didactic work was a simplified version of the medical school curriculum. It included anatomy, physiology, pharmacology, concepts of disease, medical diagnosis, physical diagnosis, and so forth.

The clinical work did not include any of the component clinical disciplines, such as surgery, medicine, paediatrics, psychiatry, and so forth.

It was hoped that the product would have the flexibility and the background to work in most medical settings and that he would have an adequate background for future learning as more specific training was required.

Early in the programme we were faced with the choice of styles of practice for this new individual: independence from, or dependence on, the doctor. We elected for dependence, meaning that the assistant depends on the doctor for diagnosis and a prescription of treatment. The assistant collects the historical data, physical data, and laboratory data needed for the diagnosis. He is also the person who often carries out the prescribed treatment under the physician's direction. There is a requirement that the doctor be a component within the system, in that the information is fed to the doctor and the prescription or plan is fed back to the assistant in the form of further instructions.

This choice was based on the following reasoning: If one elects for independence, then the current procedures for licensure will require that the assistant's permitted tasks be specified and described in great detail as a part of the law within the particular state or area in which the assistant is working.

This is a political fact in the USA. These laws are specific and are quite tightly regulated. They are also designed state-by-state, and there is no national uniformity. We therefore felt that the *dependent* mode of action —in which the specification of tasks is not by law or by description in the statute but is the responsibility of the employing doctor—would create a more flexible system and allow continued growth, both in type of tasks performed and in degree of responsibility allowed. The paradox is that a dependent role is, in the end, a less restrictive and rigid system than an independent role.

Thus, assistants are trained to perform those tasks which lead to a diagnosis and to carry out indicated treatment procedures, but it is understood that they function under the authority and under the responsibility of the employing doctor.

It is also understood that an assistant works for an individual doctor or a small group of doctors, not an institution. For example, he does not work for a hospital. His salary could come from the hospital; but one individual, one doctor within that hospital, is designated as the responsible supervising physician, and the responsibility rests with him.

I would emphasize parenthetically that this responsibility is not only a *moral* responsibility but is a *legal* responsibility as well.

I have already mentioned that the first trainees in the programme were military hospital corpsmen with experience in patient care, but I should be more specific about the requirements for selection.

In the early days of the programme, the first requirement was that the candidate have at least one or two years experience of direct patient care. We next required that there be a minimum of a high (secondary) school education. Most of the trainees, even at the beginning, had some college experience. From the outset, much emphasis was placed on the candidate's reliability and acceptance of responsibility in his previous work environment. Considerable attention was directed toward previous work experience and recommendations from previous employers.

The selection procedure has since been slightly modified. We still require previous health care experience, and we still emphasize that reliability and responsibility, as well as empathy for the patient, must be clearly demonstrated by previous experience and by letters of recommendation from previous employers. Many of the applicants are still from the military world, but an increasing number are from civilian backgrounds. We now require that the applicant have one college-level course in biology and one college-level course in chemistry before entering the programme. In many cases these courses are obtained in the summer prior to entry into the programme, after acceptance is assured.

As time has passed, a still greater percentage of applicants have had previous college experience, and a substantial number, now about one-half, already possess a baccalaureate degree. We review grades, recommendations, and college board examination scores, and narrow out the number of applicants to about twice the number that will be accepted into the programme. They are interviewed by four to six faculty members, and a final selection is made on the basis of personal interviews.

The total number of applicants each year for this particular programme at Duke University is usually about 1000 for 40 positions. The first class consisted of three students; the second class, five students; the third, twelve; and so forth. We now accept 40 students in each class. Thus, we have 80 in training in our two-year programme.

Until now, we have graduated 108 physician's assistants (or PAs), and these are widely scattered over the USA. A second point is that they are in all types of medical practice, from rural general practices to urban specialty groups.

Since our programme was the first of its kind in the USA, many of our graduates have been employed by other training programmes started in more recent years. Fifteen graduates are so employed. On the map there is a cluster of triangles in Oklahoma, many of which represent graduates associated with the University of Oklahoma programme. Other clusters in Houston, Texas, and Iowa City, Iowa, represent the same pheno-menon.

On 1 March 1973, there were 55 graduates employed in general or primary medical care settings, and 26 in specialty settings. The latter were working with paediatricians, surgeons, ophthalmologists, and so forth. In nine instances there is incomplete information regarding the exact type of practice in which the assistant is employed. Three were in transition from one position to another and were thus unemployed at that time.

There are now a number of other programmes training similar types of assistants. In September 1972, the American Medical Association report-ed that there were 72 programmes training physician's assistants, of which 29 were training individuals in the area of primary care or general medical care. Twenty-one of these 29 programmes were physician's assistant programmes, similar to the Duke programme, and eight were MEDEX-type programmes, which will be described later. Thirty-four programmes were training primarily for specialty work, such as ortho-paedics, paediatrics, psychiatry, surgery, and so forth. Four programmes were training both general and specialized assistants. There were five Federal programmes training physician's assistants for governmental service, mostly branches of military service.

Let me comment briefly on the reception that this programme has received from 1966 to date. First, the medical reaction has been mixed but generally favourable. The most favourable opinions have come from those who had the greatest need for assistance, the doctors in rural and urban deprived areas. The most reticent were doctors in areas of relative affluence in terms of medical manpower.

Most surveys have shown that a majority of doctors in the USA are in favour of this new type of manpower, but that a substantial number are opposed to it as a threat to the quality of medical care or to the role of the doctor.

Reactions from the nursing profession were also mixed but were even more adverse than those from medicine. One reason for this state of affairs was some very early publicity in which a headline writer placed the physician's assistant role above that of the nurse.

As time has passed, acceptance within organized nursing has become more frequent and more open. In my opinion, the physician's assistant movement has opened new opportunities for nurses as well, and this has become recognized and helped to mend the breach. At Duke University, our relationships with our own School of Nursing are very cordial, and we work together on joint programmes and projects which have led to greater opportunities for the nursing student as she progresses through nursing school.

One question that always arises is that of legal status. The medical and nursing professions are among the more tightly regulated professions in our culture; it is not surprising, therefore, that legal questions arise with respect to this new type of health manpower.

As with the acceptance of physician's assistants by physicians themselves, the acceptance by the state legislatures has not been uniform. At present, 27 states have recognized the physician's assistant movement by passing specific forms of legislation which would accommodate the activities of physician's assistants within their terms. In eight states specific legislation has been introduced and defeated. In the remainder of the states, there has been no action one way or another. In many of the latter, physician's assistants are working without specific legislative authority.

Next, I would like to comment on the impact of the physician's assistant on the process of medical practice, particularly with respect to patient acceptance and output of services.

We have had experience with the physician's assistant for about seven years. From the beginning, we have deliberately introduced this new type of health worker into settings in which there could be no suggestion of an inferior grade of medical care. We have utilized him, for example, in medical care for our own university faculty. In our faculty health clinic, the first medical person who contacts the faculty member is a physician's assistant who establishes the initial history and performs the physical examination. He then introduces the patient to the doctor for further review of data, for further examination, and for decisions.

In only one or two instances has the patient refused the services of the physician's assistant. In almost all instances, patients have accepted this arrangement without reluctance.

This has generally been true in other practice settings over the country. As long as the patient is aware of the fact that the physician's assistant is a part of the doctor's team, the assistant is accepted in the same fashion as the laboratory technologist, the X-ray technologist, and other members of the office team.

The impact of the assistant on the output of work from a given practice or setting has also been fairly uniform. In the analyses to date, the output has been increased by 50 to 75%.

The potential increase in output is not always fully utilized by the physician. For example, the physician may be working 12 to 14 hours a day, and rather than see more patients he may choose to have more time away from his practice. Thus, the increased capacity is used to provide more leisure rather than more units of service.

Task analyses have been done, and the results have been incorporated in the programme. Analyses of the work of a physician's assistant trained by the programme as he goes into a practice setting have been especially useful. We have learned that it is quite important for the doctor to learn to use the physician's assistant. There are examples in which the addition of a physician's assistant has made no change in the pattern of patient care by the doctor himself. This is not a desirable situation. The physician should change his pattern of care with the acquisition of a physician's assistant. He should reserve his time for more complex problems and should delegate the more routine and less complex problems to his assistant. This does not always occur, and we feel that this is a fault of medical education, not physician's assistant education.

Task analyses have also shown that minor surgical tasks such as the treatment of lacerations, abrasions, and minor trauma are often delegated to the assistant, because they are time-consuming and can be performed by the physician's assistant with great skill. We are now incorporating this information into the training programme and giving all our assistants more ambulatory surgical training.

There are always a variety of unresolved issues with any new programme, and even after seven years we still have a lot of problems. The problem of dependence and independence is one. I have indicated that our assistants are trained as dependent assistants, but at the same time we realize that the greatest need for such individuals lies in areas where there are no doctors at present. How can this be accommodated?

The next logical question is: What is dependence, and what is independence? We have only to look at the astronauts in their satellite to realize they are quite a distance from the earth, and yet they are totally dependent on the earth for decisions, supervision, and so forth.

The point that I am making here is that physical distance does not necessarily affect the question of dependence or independence. There are a number of ways in which dependence can be maintained over a long geographical span. One method of augmentation, or extension, of dependence is by standing orders or protocols, which are now being utilized in a number of settings for the control of dependent assistants. These are simply orders which specify what the assistant should do under certain circumstances. If these orders do not fit the circumstances, then the assistant cannot act.

The second method, which is under consideration but has been tried in only a few locations, is the use of technical devices such as television, radio, and so forth. These methods also seem to have some promise.

It seems, then, that there may be ways to resolve the issue of dependence and independence in very isolated areas. One of our trainees currently operates in a very remote area, a long distance from his medical supervisor, but under a system of standing orders.

Another, but quite different, problem is that of the length of time needed to train a physician's assistant. As time passes, there is pressure, primarily from educators, for a greater formalization of the educational process. This could result in extending the programme, a month at a time, to the point where it approaches the length of the medical school curriculum. As medical curricula are shortened, it is possible that the two will require similar spans of time.

I do not think that an increase in the length of the educational process is required or indicated in the case of the physician's assistant; indeed, there are training programmes that require a much shorter period of training than does our particular programme.

Another problem is the tendency for physician's assistants to be monopolized by the medical and surgical specialties. In this country, specialty practice often has economic advantages over general or non-specialty practice. This means that the specialist is often able to outbid the family physician seeking the services of a physician's assistant. As I said above, 25 of our trainees are now working with specialists. We did not direct our graduates into these areas, but in the USA there can be no compulsion to enter a particular type of practice. Assistants can go anywhere they wish and into any type of practice they like. They go to a location which meets their desires and in which their skills are remunerated to the best advantage.

This is not all bad, since specialists also need help; nevertheless, we need a more effective way to induce assistants to work with those who need them most rather than with those who need them least.

There are also unresolved problems in the area of regulation of the physician's assistant. Regulation and licensure are always legal matters under the control of each state government. Every state enjoys independence in this respect. There is a great need for some form of national certification, or some national examination that could be taken by assistants, which could be used by the individual states and which could form a basis for some form of national accrediting or national certification of the degree and type of training.

Another problem that has been raised is that of professionalization within the ranks of the physician's assistants. Some critics of such programmes feel that this new manpower category will naturally develop into a new professional group that will seek and fight for its own identity and independence. These critics feel that it could thus evolve into a second level of medical manpower. If this should occur, I would personally consider it a failure on the part of doctors to incorporate the physician's assistant correctly into the health care system.

What educational lessons have we learned from the programme over the past seven years? As for the process of training, the most important lesson is that the teaching must be done by medically trained faculty. Even the basic science courses must be taught by those who know which segments of the discipline are of particular relevance to the assistant. A field such as physiology must be taught with rare skill and selectivity in order to cover the relevant concepts within the unusually tight time schedule imposed by this programme. This is not a task to delegate to the newest graduate student in physiology; it is one for a person with knowledge of the field and with an interest in this particular form of teaching.

Clinical teaching must be done by the same techniques that are employed in teaching medical students. The same instructor–student ratios and the same number of hours are needed to learn a topic such as physical diagnosis. We have found no real short cuts in this area.

The requirement of many hours of physician teaching time dictates that almost all physician's assistant training programmes must exist in university training centres. This puts another burden on an already overtaxed system which is trying its best to increase the output of physician manpower as well.

I must emphasize, however, that medical faculty members who have had experience in teaching both medical students and physician's assistants find that the satisfactions of teaching the two groups are the same. technical skills, such as auscultation, palpation, suturing, etc., are learned with equal speed and thoroughness by the physician candidate and by the physician's assistant candidate.

The degree to which the taking of an excellent medical history and the performance of a physical examination can be mastered, and the excellence of the verbal presentation and the written chart produced by the physician's assistants (and nurse practitioners as well), often surprise the uninitiated physician. Some assistants are capable of producing charts which cannot be distinguished from those prepared by physicians.

Another fact that I would like to emphasize is that the education of the physician's assistant, like that of the doctor, is never complete. The assistant has a very important learning task as he begins to work with a new practitioner. He must become familiar with the practitioner's techniques, preferences, and idiosyncrasies. Later, the assistant must also keep abreast of medical advances. Postgraduate education is best obtained through the same courses and the same teaching exercises undertaken by physicians themselves, and not in separate sessions.

As has already been implied, some doctors can never master the art of delegation. They cannot assign tasks to anyone else and hence they cannot effectively utilize a physician's assistant.

Others are not willing to accept the obligation to become familiar with the assistant's capabilities and to recognize his skills. Each doctor must be thoroughly familiar with his own assistant's assets and limitations.

We are occasionally asked whether we have objective evidence of the effect of a physician's assistant on the quality of care in a given practice. My answer is that we have about as little information about quality of care in these settings as we do about the quality of care that is delivered by doctors in general. We have very imperfect tools with which ito measure the quality of care and the ultimate impact of this care on the future health and development of an individual. I have the feeling that those practices which are utilizing physician's assistants are delivering a higher quality of service than their counterparts without such assistants, mainly because there is some educational interplay between doctor and assistant. There is also an evident *esprit de corps* in these practices. They are proud of the fact that they are utilizing something new, and they are probably more inclined to keep up with the state of the art, since they are being observed more closely.

I would like to close by stating that the physician's assistant will be an important, and even essential, component of health care in the USA and in other countries in the future.

With proper responsibility and supervision, the services delivered by the physician's assistant can be equal in quality to those delivered by the doctor himself, and the result of this activity can be equally as effective as the traditional system in which all services are done by the doctor. The economic and other advantages must be realized and full and effective use made of them.

NURSE PRACTITIONER, CHILD HEALTH ASSOCIATE, AND PRIMARY-CARE MEDICAL PRACTITIONER

by HENRY K. SILVER, M.D.[1]

I would like to share with you our experiences of the past and our plans for the future. All of them are appropriate and pertinent to the present conference.

All here agree that there is a shortage of professionals to provide health care. If we look at this situation carefully, we will also agree that the shortage can be met in only one way—by preparing health professionals other than doctors to provide the health care that is needed.

A number of solutions have been recommended. It has been suggested that we enlarge existing schools of medicine, start new schools of medicine, shorten the training period for medical students, increase the efficiency of practising physicians, and make use of technology such as television and the computer. However, none of these are sufficiently practical and inexpensive to meet our present needs. Our basic requirement is for new health professionals.

I would like to describe for you three of the programmes developed at the University of Colorado to prepare new categories of health professionals, and to tell you of still another new programme that will be started in the near future.

Each of our health professionals is capable of a high degree of decision-making and can practise with considerable independence. He serves as an associate of the physician rather than as an assistant. We might describe the associate as someone with the capability of independent practice and decision-making comparable to that of the physician. In contrast, the assistant is someone in a much more dependent position who acts as a medical technician. In a classification of this type, an aid would be someone who has received on-the-job training or a minimum of formal training and merely carries out tasks that are prescribed by the physician.

The first health professional trained to serve as an associate of the physician in the 1960s was graduated from our programme in 1965. She is the paediatric nurse practitioner. There are now approximately 150

[1] University of Colorado Medical Center, Denver, Colorado.

graduates from the programme and altogether between 800 and 1000 practising throughout the USA.

In the paediatric nurse practitioner programme, graduate nurses receive four months of training that enables them to fill a greatly expanded and improved role in providing direct patient care to children. The nurses who enter this programme may or may not have a baccalaureate degree. They learn how to take a medical history, perform a complete medical physical examination, perform and interpret various laboratory tests and procedures, become efficient in setting up and modifying plans for immunization, and become highly skilled in preventive paediatrics. They provide excellent care to newborn infants and manage the health care of almost all well children; under a physician's standing orders they also provide extensive care to those who are ill or injured.

The four-month programme at the medical centre includes a moderate amount of didactic teaching and a large amount of practical experience of patient care in a variety of clinical settings such as nurseries, clinics, outpatient departments, and paediatricians' offices. On completion of the course at our medical centre, they have the skill, ability, and competence to care for approximately three-fourths of the children seen in various ambulatory settings. They can provide comprehensive health care to these children and do so without supervision. Some of our nurse practitioners have operated at considerable distances from physicians, with physician supervision for only half a day a week or less. For the remainder of the time they were on their own. Despite this, they provided excellent care to the children they saw.

Paediatric nurse practitioners are very well accepted by all socio-economic groups. We found that in the offices of private paediatricians they were accepted by 95% of the patients and parents. Of interest was the finding that more than half of the patients felt that the care given to them jointly by paediatricians and paediatric nurse practitioners was better than the care they had received from the paediatrician alone.

Utilization of paediatric nurse practitioners not only increases the number of children who can obtain adequate health care but also improves the level of health care that is provided.

We have carried out a number of evaluation studies on these nurses. In one study involving some 185 children, we found that the nurses' ability to assess the children's clinical condition was comparable to that of the physicians. In only about 1% of all cases was a significant difference in assessment noticed. In one of the two cases, the physician was correct; in the other the nurse was right. In this study the children presented the full spectrum of conditions ordinarily seen in a physician's office.

In the past eight or nine years, we have shown quite clearly that the four-month course given to graduate nurses can prepare them to give extensive health care to a large percentage of children seen in ambulatory settings. This is a very rapid and inexpensive way of preparing the health professionals we need.

Many of you come from countries that have appreciable numbers of nurses who are not in practice. Expanding the role of the nurse as I have described often acts as a stimulus to bring nurses back into active practice and brings greater satisfaction to those who are in practice.

We have long recommended and are beginning to see the incorporation of paediatric nurse practitioner concepts into the undergraduate nursing curriculum. These concepts, when applied in practice, make it easier for the nurse to do what she came into nursing to do—namely, to have a nursing role that is challenging, that permits her to provide the best patient care, and allows her to be a nurse in the finest sense of the word. It also permits the physician to do what he was trained to do.

Many physicians are dissatisfied with the so-called 'routine' care that they provide to patients. This is often an area that gives great satisfaction to nurses and, as a result, they often can give better care to these patients than physicians can. The physician then can do the things that he finds more challenging and satisfying.

Several years ago I made the prediction that if 100 nurse practitioner programmes were developed in the USA, we would be able to double the amount of health care provided to children. Since approximately 45 such programmes have now been established, we are already nearly half way toward that goal. In other countries, also, similar programmes could certainly improve the health care given to children.

A second type of health professional trained at our medical centre is the child health associate. This programme was started because we wanted health professionals who were even better than paediatric nurse practitioners in giving health care to children.

The child health associate programme is unique in the USA. Students entering the programme have had two years of preparation in a college or university. We then give them a three-year course with the main emphasis on paediatrics. On completion of the five years of training they are qualified to work with physicians, either in public health facilities or in their offices. Child health associates can care for approximately 90% of the patients that go to paediatricians' offices.

In the first of the two years at the medical centre, the emphasis is on the basic sciences. The students take anatomy, biochemistry, physiology, pathology, pharmacology, and almost all the other courses taken by medical students. Aspects of these courses that deal with other specialties are largely eliminated.

Child health associate students spend more time on, and get more experience of, the health care of children as applied in ambulatory settings than do medical students in medical school or most paediatric house staffs. Child health associates learn about the care of well children as well as preventive paediatrics, the care of children with minor problems, counselling, and other aspects of patient care.

We have compared the knowledge of the basic sciences and the clinical competence of child health associate students with those of medical students and members of paediatric house staffs. If the same examination is given to medical students and child health associate students, and the examination is limited to paediatrics, both groups do almost equally well. Although residents do better on clinical examinations, the performance of child health associates is entirely satisfactory.

It is of more importance to determine how child health associates perform in actual clinical situations. We have done this by comparing diagnostic abilities in approximately 150 instances where children were examined both by child health associates and by paediatricians. The same diagnosis or diagnoses were made in 93 % of the cases. In approximately 3 %, the child health associates made diagnoses that had not been recorded by the paediatrician; in 3 %, the paediatrician made a diagnosis missed by the child health associate. In no instance was the difference a significant and major one. Thus, we have evidence that the clinical competence of child health associates is entirely satisfactory.

In conformity with the law governing the practice of child health associates in Colorado, they may make medical diagnoses, institute medical therapy, prescribe a large variety of drugs, and write prescriptions. Only narcotic drugs and a few other prohibited ones are unavailable to them, and these are not particularly important in paediatrics.

Graduates of our programme serve as employees of physicians, but in that capacity they have considerable independence although they are under the ultimate supervision of the employing doctor. We feel that some degree of supervision is a necessary and desirable restriction in that it maintains adequate control of the practice of the child health associate.

Some have claimed that Colorado's child health associate law is restrictive because it defines the supervisory role of the physician. We feel that the law is very permissive because it allows the graduate child health associate to diagnose, treat, and write prescriptions. Thus, child health associates are allowed to do most of the things which a physician does in an office setting.

Students entering our programme after a minimum of two years of college preparation earn a baccalaureate degree following the first two years in the programme. Those who enter with three or more years of preparation are eligible for a master of science degree, which they earn at the end of the three-year training programme. The child health associate programme is the only one that awards both a baccalaureate and a master's degree.

In order to qualify for practice, graduates must pass an examination administered by the Colorado State Board of Examiners. We have given this examination to medical students and paediatric house staff. Child health associates made better grades than did medical students, while paediatric residents performed better than the other two groups.

According to the Colorado law, child health associates must continue their education following graduation and provide evidence that they have participated in a particular number of hours of continuing education.

Now that the child health associate programme is in operation, we find that it is considerably less expensive to prepare the associate for practice than is the case for general practitioners or paediatricians.

Child health associates have great potential for the future. Most of them work in public health facilities with medically deprived children. A number of them are practising in rural areas that have not had adequate medical coverage. They are employed both by general practitioners and paediatricians.

The third health professional programme that we developed is the school nurse practitioner programme. This was developed to improve the ability of school nurses to provide health care to school-age children. In the USA there are approximately 20 000 school nurses. On the whole, the health care they provide is neither very intensive nor extensive. We feel that the school setting, where children between the ages of 5 and 16 to 18 can be seen regularly, is one of the best places for providing health care. If competent health professionals are available, they can give a great deal of the health care that these children require.

In the school nurse practitioner programme, graduate nurses (who have frequently had experience as school nurses) come to our medical centre for a four-month course. They learn many of the things that are taught to the paediatric nurse practitioners, but the emphasis is on those skills that will be of greatest value in the school setting. In this programme, too, they do many of the things previously considered the prerogative of physicians; they also have many functions and activities that are not performed by anyone.

In the USA, many children have learning problems, psychomotor disorders, behaviour difficulties, and perceptual problems. These are not acute in most instances and, unfortunately, many children with these conditions that significantly interfere with learning never reach a physician for care. Even if they do see a physician, the follow-up is often inadequate. It is in dealing with such problems and in providing adequate follow-up care for other disturbances that the school nurse practitioner has particular value.

In comparing school nurse practitioners with 'regular' school nurses, we found that the former do many things not done by school nurses. Nurse practitioners can handle more problems on their own, need to refer fewer children for additional assessment and care, and are able to explain problems to parents in such a way that required follow-up is more likely to occur.

Most school nurse practitioners serve in areas where the numbers of doctors are grossly inadequate and children do not receive the medical care they require. As a result of their ready availability, more children are able to remain in school and those who are ill are able to return to class more quickly. In addition, their presence produces a monetary saving to the school system. School nurse practitioners have an economic value as well as a medical value for the community.

The last programme I would like to describe is one that is being developed at present to prepare a health professional whom we are calling the primary-care medical practitioner. We plan to graduate these health workers within five years after graduation from high school. They will be prepared to provide independent, autonomous primary care limited to one area of medicine. They will be largely restricted to caring for ambulatory patients, although some degree of hospital care will be permissible. Some primary-care medical practitioners will limit themselves to the health care of children; others will be concerned principally with obstetrics; still others might be concerned with geriatrics or some other specialty. Although they will be independent, autonomous practitioners, they will not have to have a doctorate degree.

The model for the primary-care medical practitioner is the child health associate programme in which the emphasis in the first year is on the basic sciences, in the second year on clinical paediatrics, while the third year consists of an internship with experience in a number of ambulatory and hospital settings. The primary-care medical practitioner will follow courses similar to those of the child health associate. They, also, will be prepared for practice five years after graduation from high school. This is only slightly more than half the training given to general practitioners and less than half that of paediatricians. Although it is expected that initially the trainees will limit themselves to one area of medicine, in time we will determine whether a similar programme covering a more general practice would be possible.

On completion of our programme, primary-care medical practitioners would be allowed to practise by themselves, but it would be expected that physicians who have doctorate of medicine degrees would serve as their consultants and advisers.

The primary-care medical practitioner programme is now in the planning stage, but on the basis of our experience with the child health associate programme we can say with a fair degree of assurance that our aims for the former can be met.

Although the time necessary to train primary-care medical practitioners may be only half as long as that necessary to prepare medical doctors, the former will have more experience than medical students of the types of patients and conditions that they will encounter in their practices.

Personally, I feel that students who take an abbreviated medical curriculum of four, five, or even six years should not be awarded a doctorate of medicine degree. This degree should be reserved for those students whose education provides them with special skills, training, and knowledge. Medical doctors should be scientists, specialists. On the other hand, primary-care medical practitioners could be prepared in a relatively short time, since their abilities can be applied to a restricted area of medicine practised primarily in ambulatory settings.

We feel that the training of primary-care medical practitioners should be given in a medical school setting and that they should be considered as another type of physician-student, even though they are not aiming for a doctorate degree. We do not feel that separate schools should be established for them. A further advantage from having primary-care medical practitioners in medical schools is that the two groups of students can learn to work together in providing health care to patients.

Primary-care medical practitioners will serve as personal physicians for patients and will be the patient's first contact with the health care system. They will be able to provide comprehensive care for most patients and will be able to recognize any serious conditions in others and refer them as necessary. Although the overall supervision of primary-care medical practitioners would be the responsibility of doctors of medicine, this would not apply to the immediate supervision of individual patients.

Primary-care medical practitioners could furnish the major portion of health care, and they could be the key figures in the health care system. On the basis of our experience with the child health associate programme, we are certain that the primary-care medical practitioner would be a very competent and effective professional health worker.

In conclusion, I would like to describe a project we are developing for people from other countries who might wish to come to our medical centre to learn how our various allied health professional programmes function and the necessary requirements for establishing similar programmes in their own countries. They would come to our medical centre for a nine-month period during which they would participate in all parts of our programmes, including administration, student teaching, and all aspects of practice of the various categories of graduates. We feel that this would be a very valuable experience. When they return home they could establish educational programmes, designed for the particular needs of their countries, that would train health professionals for the specific tasks and duties they were expected to perform. Thus individual workers would be more likely to remain where they were needed.

One of the most important things that could be done in the area of health care is to realign the role of various health professionals and to encourage greater acceptance by other health professionals of the expanded role of each. Many of the boundaries and restrictions that have separated various professions are quite artificial and unnecessary. To provide optimum and maximum health care, we need to prepare people who are competent to give the type of health care that is required in a particular setting, irrespective of the length of training. We need to overcome the resistance that various established health professionals now show towards the idea of change, and to allow each health professional to develop his professional skills to the maximum.

MEDEX

by *RICHARD A. SMITH, M.D., M.P.H.*[1]

The need to improve and to expand primary or basic health services is a subject to which many of us in the field of international health have given much attention. In late 1968, a decision was made to try a new approach to the problem. The aim was to develop a new image of a competent provider of basic health services who would complement and extend the capacity of practising doctors. This involved devising a system of training for this new kind of health manpower and deploying it into areas of need.

It was not to be a simple training programme but rather a training and deployment system, adaptable to the needs of diversified social and cultural groups in varying geographical locations. We studied health services and manpower development programmes in numerous countries of Africa, Asia, Europe, and North and South America, paying attention to their strengths and their weaknesses. From this analysis, we intended to develop a system that circumvented as much as possible the major problems of manpower development programmes.

I refer to problems such as inappropriate training and overtraining for the tasks to be performed in a particular area, identification before training of opportunities for employment in areas of great need, maldistribution, proper supervision, competition with doctors, problems of the identity and the image of a new health services provider, community acceptance, high capital investment, long periods of training and lack of significant faculty and facilities for training. These were all matters for consideration as the MEDEX concept was being developed.

The system of training and deploying MEDEX, as this new provider of health services is called, is now in operation in 30 states, including remote areas of Alaska. In addition, MEDEX are being trained to provide primary health services to populations in the distant Pacific islands of Micronesia, approximately 4000 miles southwest of Hawaii. The image of such health services being provided only by physicians is being changed both in America and in other parts of the world.

---

[1] University of Hawaii, School of Medicine, Honolulu, Hawaii.

MEDEX is a systematic way of increasing the quantity of health services provided to a larger number of people in a relatively short time. In discussing MEDEX, it is important to understand the connotation of the name. What we wanted to do was invent a simple name that could be used as a title and form of address and would not be encumbered with a lot of history. It is at once a programme and a person. It is a refinement of earlier health manpower development experience in numerous countries. And its basic elements can be applied with relatively little capital investment. We have found that it can then be continued, with modest maintenance expenditure, until the desired level of medical care accessibility is reached.

MEDEX has characteristics that make it adaptable, as opposed to transplantable, to many areas. It uses only the human and financial resources already available in the area, and it trains health manpower appropriate to the specific needs of a community. MEDEX became integrated into present health systems by extending the reach of physicians, rather than substituting for them. This is a game of semantics, but represents also a conceptual factor that must be appreciated to avoid alienation of health professionals, such as our own colleagues in the medical profession, who must also take part in planning for such an innovation.

In the USA, former medical corpsmen as well as nurses are being trained as MEDEX. Micronesia's MEDEX are former nurses and health assistants. Individuals with or without previous health backgrounds can be trained to become physician extenders when the MEDEX concept is used to improve the delivery of health services in various areas.

The MEDEX programme was initiated in 1969 without publicity. That was part of our strategy. In fact, the system was duplicated in two other medical schools before the news media began publicizing the general acceptance by Americans of someone other than physicians as providers of primary health services. The physician's assistant and the nurse practitioner were already being accepted about that time as providers of health services, so the idea was not entirely new.

There are now centres for MEDEX in three-fifths of the states of the USA. All of the MEDEX programmes are built upon six basic elements, which I shall describe. At present, about half of the medical assistants who are certified and in practice in the country are MEDEX, and about 98 % of them are working in primary or basic health care delivery, or what may be called family health services.

The reasons for the emergence of a system such as MEDEX were stated in part last year at the First International Conference on Education in the Health Sciences, held in The Hague, Netherlands. Dr Bror Rexed, head of the Swedish health system, described some of the pressures for change in medical and health services. Among them were increasing cost, the expension of demand for ambulatory care, and the introduction of new technology.

In a recent book,[1] Professor Isador Gordon points up the problems of trying to train only traditional categories of health professionals. He states that present efforts to meet the global crisis in health care solely by training more physicians are likely to fail. I believe we must continue to train increasing numbers of physicians, as well as nurses and other health professionals; but in order to increase their efficiency and enable them to cover larger geographical areas, we must now begin taking steps which would not have been considered only a few years ago.

MEDEX was developed to meet the need to extend health services against the background described by Rexed and Gordon. It is also a response to the call by Fendall and others to take much of the knowledge accumulated through research in medicine and other fields and apply it in the countries where the greatest need exists.

Using applied research methods, the MEDEX system to increase primary health services has been made flexible; it has six basic elements that are adaptable as dictated by local needs and resources.

To demonstrate that these six basic elements of the MEDEX system can be adapted—and I continue to use the term 'adapted' rather than 'transplanted'—to a less developed setting, the University of Hawaii has initiated a MEDEX programme in collaboration with the Government of Micronesia in the Trust Territory of the Pacific Islands. The training programme is based in the Truk Lagoon which covers some 3 million square miles, 92 inhabited islands, and a population of about 100 000.

Like the American MEDEX programmes, it consists of an intensive three-month didactic training phase, followed by a nine-month preceptorship or on-the-job training with a practising physician. That project also is being funded by the Bureau of Health Resources Development of the Department of Health, Education, and Welfare, and it is providing health services to some of the most isolated populations of the world.

In Micronesia, as in many parts of the USA, MEDEX are delivering services while separated from their supervising doctor by distances of 20 to 500 miles. These are what we call supervised remote practices, or SRP's. I think you understand why we have to talk about supervised remote practices rather than independent duty, especially in this part of the world. These same sensitivities may exist elsewhere. One advantage of the flexibility of this approach is that health services can be delivered where they are needed in remote and isolated areas.

The Micronesian Government, in this matter following the opinion of the United Nations Council on Trusteeships, considers this approach to provide a firm basis upon which to develop a relatively inexpensive, expanded health service providing quality care to a larger number of people, particularly in rural areas. To adapt this MEDEX concept to a country with very few doctors required a change in the one-to-one relationship of physician to MEDEX that we have here in the United

[1] Gordon, I., ed. (1971) *World health manpower shortage: 1971–2000*, Durban, Butterworth.

States. In Micronesia, a physician may be supervising two or more MEDEX who are located some distance away from him. This multiplier effect, or extensions of the doctor, is an obvious adaptation of this essentially non-complex health manpower system.

The first of the six basic elements referred to above is the collaborative model. To obtain as much information as possible regarding the possible reasons a programme may not work, as well as the ways to make it work, groups with a vested interest in making health activities more efficient and responsive to the needs of society are brought together at the beginning of the programme. These groups include professionals at the top of the health hourglass, whose control of the field should not be threatened, as well as representatives of major professional organizations and organizations only marginally involved with the new paraprofessional. They are encouraged to work cooperatively rather than competitively towards imperative common goals.

An essential element in this collaboration must be a respected medical training institution, preferably a medical school or teaching hospital. It serves three major functions:

(a) To provide quality academic input during a relatively short academic training phase;
(b) To provide programme stability and certification of professional competence;
(c) To provide the essential credibility required to instil confidence in the MEDEX's work as viewed by his or her supervisor or employer, the highly trained doctor, and the consumer of his services, the public.

These collaborators are given the opportunity to establish programme policy, particularly if MEDEX are to work in supervised remote practices at considerable distances from the physicians to whom they are responsible.

The second of the basic elements is the receptive framework, something very frequently overlooked in the development of manpower programmes. Creation of a new health professional demands careful preparation to encourage positive acceptance by the medical profession, other health personnel, patients, and supporting systems such as hospitals, the legal profession and, where applicable, insurance companies. All groups and systems affected by the innovation are contacted and prepared to receive the MEDEX. Community preparation is a paramount consideration. The skills developed by community psychiatry are particularly useful for developing this very necessary receptive framework. In many instances, the difference between success and failure will depend on overcoming cultural barriers. By creating an appropriate image and concurrent identity, MEDEX appears to have overcome two difficult obstacles whose importance cannot be minimized in implementing contemporary health manpower programmes.

The MEDEX do not wear white; they wear blue, so they have both a specific name and a distinctive appearance to patients and physicians and, even more important, to themselves. They know that this is the image they have to maintain and work within their limitations to maintain it.

Legal aspects must be considered and resolved to obtain a definitive legal status for MEDEX. Where applicable, malpractice insurance must be made available.

The third basic element, and one that is crucial in the MEDEX concept, is a built-in system designed to deploy graduates into geographical areas of need. This is accomplished in part by actively involving physicians in the selection of these new paraprofessionals, their training programme and their supervision when employed.

The physicians who are to be thus involved should be selected, whenever possible, from among primary-care physicians working in or near areas of need.

After an intensive didactic or academic training phase in a medical school or teaching hospital, MEDEX trainees are promptly integrated into the office, surgery clinic or hospital environment, and the bulk of their remaining training or preceptorship takes place on the job, in surroundings similar to those of their future work situations.

This mode of training, combined with knowledge of future deployment opportunities, makes it possible to select specific positions for employment and geographical areas of service before an individual begins his training, rather than after he has completed it.

The fourth basic element of MEDEX is competency-based training. By placing emphasis on development of competence to perform specific tasks, rather than on accumulation of diplomas or degrees, the training and deployment of MEDEX can be accomplished rapidly. Here, again, the image becomes paramount in promoting acceptance of this new health care provider.

An assessment of the health service needs of the community to be served is completed and specific documentation is obtained before training is initiated. A task analysis is also carried out to determine what the trainee will be doing after graduation.

The student's competences, prior training and experience at the time of entry are considered in order to avoid wasteful and discouraging retraining for skills he already possesses. For example, in the case of a nurse, a former military medical corpsman, or a health assistant, much basic content in the curriculum may be unnecessary because the trainee already has had this foundation.

By synthesizing data accumulated during the needs assessment and analysis and by taking into account the students' entry-level skills, it is possible to develop a precise curriculum that is designed to meet the primary needs of the community and to be of maximum value in the practice setting.

The length of the academic training programme can be shortened if the trainee learns only those skills which he will require in his job. This approach to curriculum development and training encourages emphasis on pragmatic or practical clinical experience suited to today's known needs. Training people for nonexistent jobs or jobs which underutilize their skills is avoided by emphasizing appropriate training.

The fifth of these basic elements is practitioner involvement. Recognizing the need for change within one's field of endeavour is the first step to achieving that change. The development of innovations such as MEDEX can succeed only if doctors act as change agents and professionals take the lead in developing paraprofessionals. That is the considered opinion of those of us who have worked with such programmes.

The fact that physicians are involved in the programme from the beginning encourages receptivity towards the newcomer. The physician actively participates in the selection and training of the student whom he will ultimately hire or supervise as a MEDEX. The physician is therefore more prudent both in the selection process and in the training of this new professional. Because of this personal interest in MEDEX, medical practitioners are more inclined to delegate some of their tasks, to share responsibilities, and to feel comfortable in so doing. Thus the programme is helped in overcoming one of its greatest obstacles.

The involvement of doctors in the preceptorship, which is the major part of MEDEX training, also relieves the staffs of medical schools and teaching hospitals of a huge teaching burden.

The last of the six basic elements is continuing professional development or continuing education. In order that MEDEX programmes may remain viable and useful to a rapidly changing society, a mechanism is included to promote continuing professional growth of the MEDEX. An ongoing programme of continuing education not only serves to fill in knowledge gaps of which the trainee himself and his professional supervisor may become aware, but is considered an essential element of the training institution and of this collaborative model. It is the promotion of the MEDEX's education in this way that makes it possible for competent personnel, even if without a degree, to extend the capacity of physicians to meet health needs.

The close relationship between the MEDEX and his preceptor or supervisor builds confidence and increases knowledge of what each is capable of doing. In most instances in the USA, they are in close contact. But with the development of supervisory remote practices where MEDEX are stationed in communities away from their preceptors, they must work in a truly independent way. However, we consider the supervision, even if remote, to be absolutely necessary. The supervisory remote practice method has been approved by at least two state medical societies.

Each of these six basic elements reflects the necessity to obviate specific, predictable difficulties.

The newer training technologies, such as algorithms, which are branching decision-making protocols, and video-tape packages have significantly reduced the time needed to train these new professionals. By taking full advantage of the existing competences of former medical corpsmen, nurses or health assistants, competency-based training need not waste time in teaching inappropriate material. Rather, it assists individuals to develop additional skills as dictated by the all-important task analysis. If students have had no previous health backgrounds, the training will, of course, take a little longer.

This approach is producing individuals who are already increasing physician efficiency by 75 to 125%. This is measured by patient visits and hours spent in practice.

McKenzie-Pollock and others have anticipated that, in supervised remote practices, MEDEX alone will adequately handle 90% of the patient problems of an outpatient clinic. Those of you who, like myself, have treated some 300 patients a day in an outpatient clinic know that the kind of care we deliver under those conditions could be improved by about 100%. This is possible because these new professionals can perform many of the routine, repetitive medical tasks that have hitherto been solely the domain of the physician but which do not require his sophisticated training and experience. MEDEX are taught which patients require referral and which do not require the exercise of a physician's intricate decision-making processes and profound diagnostic and therapeutic skills.

Last year, NBC television completed a documentary film[1] for television which portrays MEDEX from a viewpoint that is slightly different from that which I have described. We allowed it to be filmed because we wanted to have some sort of visual documentation for local county medical societies to encourage discussion among doctors who were still afraid to make this move. If we could show physicians that patients were accepting this, that doctors themselves were training MEDEX, that nurses in their offices were working very closely with MEDEX, then we would probably have a tool which would be useful in many settings.

In summary, adaptations of the MEDEX system to multiple socio-economic, cultural, and geographical settings are now occurring. MEDEX is being developed by medical care systems in both highly industrialized and less developed areas. Taking advantage of modern advances in task analysis, competency-based training, and community psychiatry, this approach to appropriate training and deployment of physician extenders to areas where they are needed is an encouraging development in health manpower in recent decades.

---

[1] MEDEX. Produced in connexion with KING-TV in Seattle, Wash., in 1971 and revised in 1972 by the Health Instructional Resources Unit of the Bio-Medical Science Complex at the University of Hawaii, Honolulu.

THE COMMUNITY HEALTH MEDIC IN
INDIAN AMERICA

by JERRY BATHKE[1]

Today I propose to discuss the community health medic and the community health medic training programme in Indian America. I cannot begin to talk about this subject, however, without first giving you a brief review of Indian America.

In the history of North America, there is a great and ancient history of the American Indian peoples. They were diverse, their livelihood was considerable and varied throughout North America. Their numbers are the subject of considerable debate. There may have been as few as 12 000 at the time of Columbus' arrival on this continent, or there may have been as many as 5 million.

That is now of less importance than the fact that over the following few hundred years there was considerable interaction of these various Indian tribes with the western world. This resulted in their gradual containment and subsequent location on what are known as Indian reservations. These were particles or parcels of land, often not necessarily the land they knew or grew up on, within which their movements were strictly limited and regulated. This produced limited opportunity, education, responsibility, and self-respect. It is a story that does not need retelling here.

Today, Indian America comprises nearly 1 million people (about 865 000 as of the 1970 census). Approximately two-thirds of this number live on or near Indian reservations.

Unemployment ranges from 45% to 80%. Housing is 80% to 85% substandard. Education is at an average of eighth grade level (primary). The suicide rate is the highest of any ethnic group in North America. Health, by the Federal Government's standards and studies, is the poorest of any group in this nation. Facilities for health care are relatively few; there are very few clinics and very few hospitals. I am sorry to report that there are only three schools for handicapped and retarded Indian children in the whole of the United States. There is only one nursing home for Indians.

The American Indian people have been referred to by other speakers in the conference. In the context of those references, the American Indians

---

[1] Executive Director, Navajo Health Authority, Window Rock, Arizona.

could be described as 'limited and specialized Federal beneficiaries of certain health care programmes.'

But what about manpower? A comparison of health manpower shows that for a national population of 210 million, there are 340 000 physicians, whereas there are only 39 American Indian physicians for a population of 800 000. Of those 39, only three are full-blooded American Indians. Only one is practising in an American Indian community.

Among 14 000 doctors of osteopathy, there are no Indians. Among the 120 000 dentists in this country, there is only one American Indian. There are 25 000 doctors of veterinary medicine in this country, with only two American Indians, 18 000 doctors of optometry, with only one American Indian, and 120 000 pharmacists, with only six American Indians. Of the nearly 2 million nurses, aids, and orderlies in this country, not even 500 are American Indians.

The barriers to the entry of American Indians into the health careers is an entirely separate subject and two full days would be needed for its presentation.

Given this general picture of American Indians today and the circumstances of their health, I wish to talk specifically about the Navajo Indians.

The Navajo nation, as you will understand, is similar to a developing nation. It occupies an area of more than 25 000 square miles or 15 million acres lying in parts of what are the states of Arizona, New Mexico, and Utah. This is a larger area than that of any one of over 20 of the states in the USA and larger than that of many nations in the world. It is the largest tribe of American Indians.

There are 135 000 Navajos living on the Navajo reservation; yet in that large land mass there is very low population density. Theirs is a very rural way of life, devoted to sheep farming. The Navajo and the other American Indian peoples have a distinct language, a distinct culture, a distinct civilization, and a distinct way of life that has been passed on to them by the Holy People, their creators. They have a religion, traditions, and ancient expectations.

Before we can begin to understand Western medicine in Indian America today, we must understand that the Navajo people have had a medicine of their own, which they still practise. It is entirely traditional but very systematic. It describes a definite procedure for what you do when you need health care or when you believe yourself to be in need of certain corrections. It is built upon an understanding of the wholeness of the universe, a harmony with the universe, a beautiful way with everything around you. And if the parts become disarranged or out of sorts with each other, then you must conduct the right ceremonies to put these parts back in place. It is built upon responsibility. It is stratified. There are levels of the herbalist, diagnostician, singer and medicine man, who ultimately cures the condition.

Everyone does only his own thing. And there is a certain period of training and development to become learned. I want to come back to this traditional health care system and expectations as I talk about the community health medic.

The Navajo Nation is more than 450 miles from east to west and about 350 miles from south to north; it lies in no less than 13 counties, three states, and three Federal regions. Roads are very sparse in this vast area and there are only 3000 miles of paved road. This allows only a couple of roads in each direction, which is a great factor in the poor quality of health care. People cannot get to health care and health care cannot get to the people.

Rainfall is limited and erodes the soil rapidly. What little rain does come is usually washed away or trapped in catchment ponds, which in turn create their own environmental hazards—stagnant water and infected water resources. Most of the water supplies come from shallow wells. This leads to one of the leading health problems—gastroenteritis and other infectious diseases associated with poor environment. The dwellings have no running water, refrigeration, or electricity. They are one-room dwellings, with an open fire in the middle, and eight people generally live in one dwelling. Horses are still used for transport although not everyone is so restricted. Most of the livelihood is rural with very little wage economy.

The annual growth of the Navajo population is approximately 4%, among the highest of any group in North America. There is a continuing high level of natality and of infant mortality compared with United States whites and non-whites. Health statistics are comparable to the American or European statistics of 100 years ago or more.

The number of Indian neonatal and postnatal deaths is extremely high. Children are usually quite healthy until they return to the home of the mother following delivery. Then their survival is precarious for the first year or two because of the adverse environmental conditions.

Some of the leading causes of death are accidents, tuberculosis, upper respiratory diseases, and suicide—clearly not the pattern found in the general American population.

Given these conditions, what is being done? The Federal Government has a programme known as the Indian Health Service, which has approximately seven hospitals and 600 beds for this large population in this vast area. There are 108 doctors, many of whom do administrative work and do not provide primary care to the Indian population.

There are a few small mission clinics and hospitals, but, for the most part, health care is very poor and very limited, despite the fact that the Indian Health Service is accomplishing near miracles with the resources available.

It is important to observe, however, that in July 1973 the doctor draft of the Federal Government ended. Therefore, there is no longer this mechanism for sending physicians to the Navajo people.

What, then, have the local people done? The local Navajo and American people undertook some planning for their future health care. There had been little or no effort to produce Indian manpower and, since their own distinct language is the only one understood by over 50% of the people, there were limited prospects of future manpower development for the American Indians. What is more, the American Indian people wanted to become self-sustaining and to determine their own future. They consequently proposed to start an American Indian medical school and other health training programmes.

A request to that effect was transferred to the then Secretary of Health, Education, and Welfare, Dr Elliott Richardson, who established a task force headed by Dr Blue Spruce. The task force reported back to the Navajo people that such plans were indeed possible and appropriate. The Navajo Health Authority was established with 25 directors of great prominence from around the world—Navajo, other Indians, and non-Indians alike. Its basic goals were to start health manpower training programmes, to assess the feasibility of an American.Indian medical school, and to foster, guide, and assist in the development of a comprehensive health care programme appropriate to the needs of the people.

The Manpower Division of the Navajo Health Authority has the responsibility to develop jobs and to plan and develop manpower programmes. It coordinates existing training programmes such as the MEDEX programme at Utah, the midwifery programme from Utah, the midwifery programme from Johns Hopkins, the Pittsburgh programme, and Project Hope, together with any other manpower training efforts that have or will become available to the Navajo people.

It is a very important responsibility to ensure that these activities meet the real needs of the people. It is also necessary to develop the additional training programmes required at all levels—continuing education, medical education, allied health manpower, and so forth.

One programme that can meet the above requirements, can accommodate the maldistribution of physicians and health manpower, and can develop manpower training for the people in that area, is the area health education centre of the Navajo Health Authority and the University of New Mexico, funded by the Bureau of Health Resources Development of the Department of Health, Education, and Welfare.

Another example of this kind of mechanism established by the Navajo people is a career lattice which makes it possible for registered nurses to return to school and become physicians, or licensed practical nurses to become registered nurses, or other health professionals who so wish to move to another level, such as the physician's assistant.

Another example is instruction in the native healing sciences to ensure that non-Indian health professionals understand the American Indian concept of and attitudes to health as well as American Indian health professionals do.

It was in this situation that the community health medic programme was developed. Its introduction among the Navajo was admittedly exploratory. It came in the midst of great distress following the knowledge that the doctor draft and potentially all sources of doctors to this people would be lost. It came from the initiative of the Navajo people through the Indian Health Service and was begun by the Indian Health Service, with Gallup, New Mexico, as the principal training location. Another comparable programme was begun at Phoenix, Arizona.

The programme, which is supervised by the Indian Health Service, the Navajo Health Authority, and the nearest medical school (the University of New Mexico) is now a two-year course with accreditation where desired at the Associate of Arts degree level with the Navajo Community College.

It begins with an intensive three-month didactic programme, followed by nine months of specific task-oriented clinical training. The first year's training is conducted at the Gallup Indian Medical Center. This is institution-based but decentralized from the nearest medical schools. The curriculum is basically of the same nature as that described by Dr Estes and Dr Smith.

The second year of training takes place in specific field placements somewhere in the Navajo Nation under the direction of a preceptor on a one-to-one basis. Graduates become certified by the successful completion of a standard examination.

Last month, the first class graduated 15 members. The second class of ten has just finished the first year. The three classes which have either graduated or are still in training are largely composed of nurses, technicians, and medical corpsmen. They are all people of the Indian population; they have a clear intention to serve those people, and they reside in Indian areas.

One of the special features of this programme is that the students are indigenous. They have lived, intend to serve, and received their training in the target area. There are a number of reasons for this.

One is the predictable anxiety concerning their acceptability by the other health professionals and by the constituent population.

Second, these people have the fullest understanding of the needs, the expectations, and the attitudes of that population, and can thus help them most.

Third, they speak the language of the people they intend to serve. Previously, a non-Indian physician required the services of an interpreter.

Fourth, the programme is task-oriented. It is designed to meet the needs of this culture. The health needs of these people are specific and somewhat different from the needs of people living in Bethesda, Maryland, or elsewhere. For example, the students are required to demonstrate competence in 652 specific skills before they can graduate, skills that are pertinent to the needs of this population and of a priority nature.

A very special feature is the decentralization of the programme. The first year is quite decentralized and removed from the medical school; the medical teachers come to the region to give the principal training. The field placement or preceptorship experience is even more removed from the school and is conducted in the local community.

Previously there had been no programme of disease prevention or health education because the Indian Health Services facilities were over-burdened by having to see sometimes 100 or 200 patients a day with only about five minutes for each patient. Now for the first time, we have a plan and some hopes of conveying health education and concepts of preventive medicine to the people.

Another special feature of this programme is teamwork. The community health medics work with the community health representative, with the environmental sanitarian, with the public health nurse, and with the physician in remote rural areas.

Another special feature is the health care delivery system.

Finally, a feature that has been widely commented upon is the acceptability of the system with respect to the traditional expectations of the people and the traditional health care delivery system characterized by stratification, certain procedures of health care, and referral to the next level of care. The physician's assistant programme, or the community health medic, as we term it, meets those ancient and traditional expectations, but not necessarily the expectations and the acceptability of Western medicine, which the American Indian people have only come to know in the last thirty or forty years. The physician's assistant programme is built upon the relationships of the community health medic with his patients, with the constituents of his area, and with the people of the area that he comes from and that he knows.

My anxieties with regard to our programme are related to many of these points. Admittedly, the programme continues to be exploratory, but there is considerable sensitivity to some of these matters.

I know that, under the circumstances, our concern regarding acceptability may be best resolved in the way we have adopted. On the other hand, what we have begun may not be successful and we may need to make adjustments. We earnestly believe, however, that the programme can be successful only through an organization jointly responsible for health care delivery and for manpower education within a culturally relevant organizational framework. Unless we bring together health education and health care delivery, we are not going to achieve the efficiency or the success that we hope for. We have developed a culturally relevant organization, we provide direct health care delivery, and we direct health manpower education.

Another important characteristic of this programme is that it is a local programme. It was designed by the Navajo people, by American Indian people. It came from the people and not from the professionals. It did not come from 'Washingdone', as the Navajo people say. It came from the roots up, and that may be one of the principal reasons for its current success and for our expectations of its long-range success.

MEDICAL ASSISTANTS IN THE USA AS VIEWED BY THE PROFESSIONS

THE PHYSICIAN'S VIEW

by *MALCOLM TODD, M.D.*[1]

We have heard about a variety of new programmes which our profession and health planners in the USA have been charged to develop. These include the MEDEX programme, the Duke University programme, Dr Silver's programme in Colorado, and also the Navajo project which certainly seems to stimulate interest among the people themselves.

One way of increasing the supply of health services in the USA has been the delegation of an increasing number of the physician's traditional functions in delivery of health care. Such an approach involves reallocating duties between the physician and various middle-level health personnel to achieve the best use of skills at each level. This often results in reducing the time required to educate individuals to perform a given health task. This reallocation of duties can take place in two ways: first, by expanding the medical service role of existing health occupations and, second, by creating and recruiting for new career roles to assist the physician.

This presentation will focus on the latter approach and specifically on the development of new types of middle-level workers, commonly termed the medical or physician's assistant.

The concept of a physician's assistant and the delegation of the physician's tasks are not really new. Physicians have been delegating tasks of all kinds to nurses and to medical office assistants for years. What *is* new is the desire to formalize the training within university medical centres to enable a new category of personnel to perform services which extend the physician's capabilities in the diagnostic and therapeutic management of patients.

The physician's assistant, as an alternative manpower resource for extending the physician's services, has become a focus of heightened attention and concern. Interest in training physician's assistants has been primarily stimulated by educators, congressmen, and government officials, and has received further impetus from efforts to utilize the skills of military medical corpsmen returning to civilian life. As a result, the past few years have seen extensive activity by educational institutions in

---

[1] American Medical Association Council on Health Manpower, Chicago, Illinois.

various parts of the USA to develop programmes to train various new physician support occupations, generically termed physician's assistants.

Recently, the American Medical Association (AMA) collaborated in compiling a list[1] of over 80 programmes for training new types of physician support occupations.

The keynote of these programmes is variety. Length of training varies from eight weeks to five years. Educational settings include medical schools and medical centres, public and private hospitals, clinics, community colleges, colleges, and universities. The prerequisites for admission vary from high-school graduation or experience as a military corpsman to possession of a baccalaureate degree. The credentials awarded vary from none to certificates or associate, baccalaureate, or higher degrees. Proposed employment settings include physicians' offices, hospitals, clinics, and emergency rooms. Job descriptions vary from general to highly specific, and functions from the purely technical to those requiring a high level of judgement.

The range of educational programmes for the physician's assistant is to some degree illustrated by the variety of names used to describe such personnel: the clinical associate, the child health associate, the community health medic, the medical services assistant, MEDEX, and the physician's associate, to name only a few.

Some programmes recruit, in addition to former military corpsmen, persons with various levels of nursing experience, experience in allied health fields or, in some cases, high-school education only. Thus educators are producing many kinds of medical workers under the generic term 'physician's assistant' to function at different levels of responsibility in a wide range of medical activities.

Although organized medicine was not involved in originating the concept of the physician's assistant, it must assume responsibility for ensuring the orderly and rational development of these new occupations if they are to become a valuable adjunct to the delivery of medical care in the USA.

In December 1970, the AMA recommended adoption of the following working definition: 'The physician's assistant is a skilled person qualified by academic and practical training to provide patient services under the supervision of a licensed physician who is responsible for the performance of that assistant.'

Thus, in our view, the mission of a physician's assistant is to carry out, under the direction and supervision of a licensed doctor, selected diagnostic and therapeutic tasks, permitting the physician to extend his services to a greater population base through more efficient use of his knowledge, skills, and abilities.

The AMA is on record as being in favour of innovation in health manpower and, hence, of the experimental development of the physician's

---

[1] American Medical Association, Department of Manpower Intelligence, & Bureau of Health Manpower Education, National Institutes of Health (1972) *Summary of training programs; physician support personnel*, Washington, D.C., Department of Health, Education, and Welfare (Publication No. NIH 73-318).

assistant. Nevertheless, a great deal of ambivalence still exists among members of the medical profession.

Physicians have expressed concern about the entire concept. Some believe that practitioners have had little to say about the development of the physician's assistant and that the impetus has come from educators, policy makers, and organizers of health services. In other words, the demand for the physician's assistant has originated from outside the medical profession itself.

Many doctors do not know how to utilize such assistants and are reluctant to delegate tasks which they have traditionally reserved for themselves or perhaps delegated to office nurses and medical assistants. Forcing doctors to delegate tasks may be viewed as making them surrender such tasks and will not achieve the objectives sought. Moreover, the success of the physician's assistant depends as much on his relationship with his supervising physician as on where he was trained or the length or character of the programme from which he graduated.

The unrecognized status of the physician's assistant continues to be a major obstacle to the delegation of tasks to him. Some surveys of physicians' attitudes have shown a discrepancy between what physicians view as tasks that could be delegated and those that they would actually delegate. One such study was conducted by the American Society of Internal Medicine.

The future viability of this occupation on a national scale is largely undetermined. Many physicians have expressed concern that if physician's assistants are produced in large numbers, they may become substitute physicians. This inevitably leads to the question, 'Would such a development not result in two levels of physicians and, inevitably, in two levels of care?'

The AMA has been working to increase the number of medical schools and to encourage more medical students to enter family practice. Success in these efforts, combined with improvements in medical school curricula, an expanded role for the nurse, raised levels of skills of existing workers such as medical assistants, and the adoption of new techniques for the screening, testing, and monitoring of patients under medical supervision, may together actually be able to meet the currently perceived needs without recourse to large numbers of physician's assistants or additional categories of physician support personnel.

Recent surveys of selected groups of physicians have revealed that while 60% of those surveyed may feel they need additional help, only 30% indicated an inclination to hire such additional help for their own practices if such help were available.

Some medical manpower experts believe that substantially more delegation is needed than physicians now permit. There are some who contend that existing laws are flexible enough to accommodate greater delegation of medical functions to unlicensed persons through the process of evolutionary changes in the pattern of medical practice. However, more than half of the states have already felt compelled to enact or propose legislation to regulate the activities of the physicians' assistant. These attempts fall into two main categories: first, an exception to the Medical Practice Act to codify the physician's legally recognized right to delegate tasks to competent allied health personnel; and second, a broadening of the powers given to the state boards of medical examiners so that they may approve physician's assistant training programmes or approve applications submitted by physicians to utilize graduates of approved programmes.

Now, most of you do not realize that we have in the USA a subject known as states' rights, and that we have no national licensure of physicians. A physician is licensed by the individual state in which he practises, although elsewhere he can obtain a licence through reciprocity between states. Thus, to make any changes to permit allied health personnel to extend the services of the physician comes within the prerogative of the states and their rights. Individual states often guard these rights with a great deal of vigilance.

Another fundamental and essentially legal issue is whether the individual physician, rather than the medical profession or the law, should decide the extent to which medical functions can be delegated to unlicensed persons.

You can be assured, however, that the medical profession has assumed responsibility for and a leadership role in ensuring an orderly and rational development for this new occupation as well as others.

The primary concern of the AMA is that services rendered by any level of medical workers be consistent with accepted standards of quality care. In regard to new and emerging categories of allied health personnel, the AMA's Council on Health Manpower works closely with medical specialty groups and other professional organizations in evaluating the need for and the functions of new categories of health manpower. Recently, the AMA House of Delegates adopted some guidelines[1] intended to assist those organizations and institutions contemplating the training and development of new forms of health manpower.

The Council believes that it cannot presume to decide unilaterally on the merits of a particular type of physician's assistant, but it must look to the potential physician employers of such assistants and the organizations representing those physicians for two things: first, for documentation on the need for and readiness to employ these individuals, and second, a detailed job description or list of functions for such personnel. Only with this kind of information can the Council make an intelligent decision as to whether the proposed new occupation is relevant to health service needs and whether the new group of applied health workers should be invited to contact the Council on Medical Education to develop educational standards or essential norms for training.

---

[1] American Medical Association, Council on Health Manpower (1972) *Guidelines for development of new health occupations*, Chicago, Ill.

The AMA, through its Council on Medical Education, not only maintains standards for medical education but also develops and maintains standards for accreditation of allied medical education programmes. It is the accrediting agency for training programmes in 22 different allied medical occupations, including the assistant to the primary care physician, the orthopaedic physician's assistant, and the urologist physician's assistant.

Second, because programmes will continue to vary significantly in curriculum content, duration, and prerequisites for admission, even with an accreditation mechanism available, the AMA Council on Health Manpower has recognized a need for physician's assistant certification as an important complement to accreditation, particularly since a substantial number of qualified candidates, at least at the outset, will not be graduates of approved programmes.

Certification is helpful to the physician employer by providing some evidence of actual or potential competence, and not leaving him to judge this solely from the education, experience, and background of each worker. Certification provides a basic assumption of competence and, from the standpoint of the worker, facilitates his employment.

The Council on Health Manpower has agreed that it would help to ensure orderly development of the physician's assistant concept if a programme were set up which, on the basis of a nationally validated proficiency examination, would grant certification to individuals of both traditional and unorthodox educational background. Accordingly, with the approval of the House of Delegates, collaboration is under way with the National Board of Medical Examiners to develop such a proficiency examination for certification of the assistant to the primary care physician.

The construction of a valid and reliable test is a complex process, but it is hoped that the certification examination will be made available before the end of 1973. Such certification by nationally recognized medical organizations will help to maintain high standards in the occupation, will provide the potential physician employer with evidence of competence and, by providing nationally recognized credentials, will enhance the career and increase the mobility of the assistant to the primary care physician.

The AMA and the American Hospital Association have for some time been studying the status of the physician's assistant in the hospital. In an effort to assist the medical staff in regulating the utilization of such assistants in the hospital, the Council on Health Manpower has developed, in conjunction with the Committee on Nursing, a statement on 'Status and Utilization of Expanding and Emerging Health Professions in Hospitals.'[1]

This statement calls for the medical staff to recommend to the governing authority the extent of functions that may be delegated to members of these emerging or expanding health professions, to determine the general

---

[1] American Medical Association (1972), Chicago, Ill.

qualifications to be required of members of each of these health professions, and to specify appropriate utilization of such personnel, based on their professional training, experience, and demonstrated competence.

Basically, there is theoretical agreement as to the efficacy of the physician's assistant concept as a means of extending physician services. However, much consideration needs to be given to questions of legal status, patient acceptance, physician acceptance, and relationships with nurses and allied health workers, before financial support is given to develop educational programmes on a wide scale. The role and function of the physician's assistant in the medical care system need to be better defined, the appropriate educational curriculum clarified, and a way found to ensure that the best standards of education and performance are maintained.

To sum up, may I say that within the profession itself the physician's assistant concept meets with mixed emotions. While many believe that there is a need and a place for physician extenders, it is no secret that many doctors in the USA are vehemently opposed to this concept. Personally, I am not one of them. Many physicians are confused by the numerous, proliferating types of assistants. Many are unsure of the legal restraints in their employment and are worried about the ultimate malpractice dilemma. Some have a fear of independence leading to a basis for a new cult, and some are outspoken in their concern about the potential development of two standards of medical care.

The AMA's Council on Health Manpower believes that the alteration of state medical practice acts to permit the use of properly trained and supervised assistants, and certification for competent graduates of accredited programmes, offer the best safeguards to the public, the medical profession, and the physician's assistant himeslf.

One final word. When a physician's assistant is employed by a doctor, the latter has a great personal responsibility. He must properly introduce his assistant to his patients, to his professional colleagues and to members of the medical staff of his hospital, and establish the correct posture of this assistant before administrators, nurses, aids, and technicians in hospitals and facilities with which he may be associated.

The position which the physician's assistant will achieve as a health manpower resource and the tasks he will perform will eventually be determined by the willingness of physicians to employ him and to delegate tasks to him.

The AMA will continue to take a leading role in guiding the development of this emerging health occupation by assuming responsibility for accreditation and certification mechanisms.

THE NURSE'S VIEW

by *LUCY CONANT, Ph.D.*[1]

I am not representing any particular nursing organization. Rather, I am speaking from my own background of experience. At the University of North Carolina at Chapel Hill, we have a family nurse practitioner or Primex programme with which I have been actively connected for the past three years. It is from this experience that I am raising some questions, issues, and possibilities.

I would like to begin with a question: Does medical assistant mean the same thing as health care personnel? The question is whether medical care is equated with health care.

Perhaps this is being too specific about the definition of terms, but I believe that people need broader types of health services than those provided by physicians alone. The physician assistant model is, as I see it, a means of assisting the physician within the model of care provided by the physician. But there are other areas or dimensions of health care which are broader than that provided by the physician. I will come back to this point later.

There is no question that physicians should have assistants. In nursing we have licensed practical nurses, nursing assistants, nursing aids, and so forth. Dentists have dental hygienists and dental assistants. Certainly, physicians need all the help they can get.

But this is only part of the total health care delivery system. My question is: Who is going to provide the other aspects of personal health care, and than how will all of these pieces fit together, relate to the physician's services, and provide a total, comprehensive type of personal health care?

Dr Barbara Bates, in her article 'Doctor and nurse: changing roles and relations',[2] presents one of the clearest descriptions of how physicians and nurses working together can complement and supplement each other's roles to provide more comprehensive personal health care. Certainly, in this country it is recognized that health care needs have not been met,

---

[1] University of North Carolina, Chapel Hill, North Carolina.
[2] Bates, B. (1970) *New Engl. J. Med.*, 283, 129–134.

particularly for certain groups of people. Physicians have been functioning over here, nurses have been functioning over there, and there is a broad area between the traditional roles of these two groups. This is the area I am concerned about; it is an area where nurses have a very real opportunity to expand their role and to fit their services more closely with physicians' services so that more people can receive comprehensive health care.

I am anxious to make the point that what many of these assistant programmes are doing in nursing—whether it is the paediatric nurse practitioner, the family nurse practitioner or others—is to make legitimate the activities that nurses have been doing for years, particularly in rural areas. Nobody was around so the nurse did the best she could. But it never became official; it never became part of an agency policy. It was frequently done out of necessity, behind closed doors, and people often pretended that it did not happen.

Since nurses were not trained for these activities, they did the best they could with physician help and learned from experience. But these activities never became part of the educational programme in nursing; they never became part of planned organizational services and policies. What we now are recognizing is that these are legitimate health care needs, whether they take place in Alaska or in Indian reservations, in a rural area or in a city, and that people need these services. In many instances, nurses are the people who are there. Since they are the largest single group of health providers, why not prepare nurses for their broader role in health care in an organized, systematic way?

There are alternative approaches, and some of them have been presented here. There are various possibilities that need to be tried out and evaluated.

At this time in the USA, the question is not whether it should be a physician's assistant, or MEDEX, or nurse practitioner. There are some settings and situations that may be particularly appropriate for one type of health care provider; others may be appropriate for other types. Certainly, there is a need for further study and evaluation before the different models are frozen into clearly defined and structured patterns.

However, what is happening at this point is very confusing both to the American public and to health professionals. But the existing flexibility does provide an opportunity to test new approaches. I think there is a need for open minds, innovation, and experiment. Certainly, we need to make some decisions and bring about some kind of clarity and organization in relation to the types of training, expectations, and roles of the people we are discussing.

The first issue I would like to raise is the danger of fragmentation of care. Does the introduction of another provider into the health care system produce increased fragmentation and complexity into the delivery of health care? This is going to depend partly on the degree of specialization. For example, in this country there are at least two programmes preparing family planning nurse practitioners. I tend to object to that because I believe that such an overly narrow, technical approach is fragmenting care. The same question may be asked about MEDEX and other groups. This is something that needs to be looked at. Too many people are providing little bits and pieces of care. Particularly in the case of primary care, this may create more confusion and a poorer quality of care than with a smaller team working effectively together.

Then there is a question of the scope of care. Do different people need different types of care? We need to look at the particular needs of particular groups, and certainly Mr Bathke's presentation of the needs of the Navajo tribe and the efforts to provide health care that will fit in with their culture and include aspects of their traditional system of care is a very good illustration.

Again, I would raise the point that some people need only the care of physicians; other people need more. We need to look at this in terms of the scope of care, as well as the quality of particular tasks, procedures and decisions. But what about the care of families, the care of people who have several health problems, the care of people who have long-term chronic diseases, and other such groups and categories?

Then there is the question of cost. One can raise very legitimate questions about the willingness and ability of society to pay for highly trained medical specialists to provide primary care. The comment has been made that to use paediatricians for the care of well babies and children is not a very economical and efficient approach. In the long run it is up to society to decide on its ability to pay for health care and for what kind of health care.

Brief mention has been made of reimbursement, and I hope this can be discussed in more detail. In some other countries, many of which have national insurance plans or national systems of health care, it may not be a problem. But in this country, reimbursement is a very real problem for all of these new health care roles, be they the physician's assistant, nurse practitioner, or some other category.

Then there are questions about the continued professional development of the individuals in these new roles. Where does the physician's assistant go? Where does the MEDEX go? What is going to be their career potential in ten years? Because of the importance of career mobility in this country, that is something that needs to be examined.

One of my particular concerns about the MEDEX programme is what happens when the particular physician the MEDEX is working with retired or dies. Can the MEDEX transfer his knowledge and skills easily to another physician, or does this become a very individualized type of relationship? One might ask if there is danger of a MEDEX becoming 'indentured' to or too dependent upon a particular physician.

We have talked a great deal about the delivery of primary care. Are these new types of health care personnel going to stay in this field or are they going to move into the specialty areas? This is something Dr Estes spoke about in terms of the Duke University physician's associate programme. I know of several instances in which some physician's assistants or physician's associates have gone on to medical school to study to become physicians. I am not sure that this is the most efficient way of providing training for the health professions.

Also, what is going to happen to those who do continue to deliver primary care, particularly in rural areas, in relation to professional isolation and the problems of supervision? Certainly, there is a tremendous necessity for continuing education on a planned, systematic basis.

It has been difficult for physicians, nurses, dentists, and others who practise in isolated areas to keep abreast of recent developments, new practices and methods of care. This may also be a special problem for physician's assistants and nurse practitioners in isolated, remote areas. The problems that I have briefly alluded to illustrate some of the risks in planning programmes and services that need to be recognized and dealt with.

Finally, there is the question of making the most effective use of the knowledge and skills of these new health care providers. There is no doubt that training programmes—whether they are nurse practitioner programmes, physician's assistant or associate programmes, or MEDEX programmes—have demonstrated that it is perfectly feasible to teach people how to provide good quality care within their sphere of responsibility in relation to the role that has been or is in the process of being developed. But are these people going to be fully utilized?

A great deal will depend upon physicians and their willingness to delegate both authority and responsibility. I do not have specific figures, but some preliminary findings in a number of places show quite wide variations in such delegation between different physicians and extender personnel. Some physicians make very effective use of these people and continue to encourage the development of their practice roles; others do not.

Also we need to examine some of our own experience in this country in terms of our willingness to utilize people with particular knowledge and skills in the health field. I am referring to our experience with nurse midwives. In many countries, nurse midwives are accepted as an integral part of the health care system. In this country we have had nurse midwives for some time. Some of the early ones received their training in England. There have been a number of nurse midwifery programmes in this country for a number of years. As far as I know, every study that has been done has demonstrated that nurse midwives were perfectly capable of providing high quality care to women having a normal type of delivery, and yet, it is only within the last two or three years that there has been any real interest and demand for them. At the same time, in many areas our infant mortality rates and maternal complications have been appalling. But nothing happened until the suddenly awakened interest in new types of health personnel finally opened the door to the possibility of making effective use of nurse midwives.

With respect to the views of nursing organizations on these new programmes, it should be recognized that organizations are inherently resistant to change and nursing organizations are no exception. Therefore, it is not reasonable to expect the American Nurses Association or the American Medical Association to lead the way in promoting them.

It is obvious from the previous presentations that different people in different places have had different ideas, have reviewed their own situations or the national situation, and then have developed and implemented a possible approach or plan, and that organizations have responded. But the initiative has not come from the professional organizations, and it should not be expected from such groups. They have a natural concern about their professional status and about the implications for their own group of any changes. However, they do respond to outside pressures and to new developments.

I wish to comment briefly on Dr Estes' statement about the nursing response to the Duke physician's assistant programme. Many nurses throughout the country were initially apprehensive as physician's assistant programmes began to develop. At the same time, there were nurses who were curious, interested, and wanted to find out more about them. In recent years, nursing participation in some of these programmes has increased. Particularly in the last five years or so, a real about-face has taken place in the nursing profession which has shown greater interest and willingness to expand its role and move into the no man's land between traditional physician practice and traditional nursing practice.

Now nurses see these new developments and programmes as a challenge. At the same time, these developments have opened up the entire area of health care and have helped to educate the public regarding new possibilities and alternative approaches. I believe that at this time nurses are able and willing to meet that challenge and to re-define and expand their role in relation to the needs of society.

A question was raised earlier about short-term and long-term aspects and implications of all of these developments. The impetus of some of these changes has until now been of a short-term character. To return to the comments of Dr Barbara Bates, there is a real potential of a long-term character because, as was said before, people need more than physicians' care. If we can work together, we can provide efficient and effective comprehensive health care to people. That is what this conference is all about.

GROUP DISCUSSIONS

ROLES FOR THE MEDICAL ASSISTANT

Chairman: THOMAS HATCH[1]

Moderator: EDWIN F. ROSINSKI, Ph.D.[2]

ROSINSKI (*USA*): Perhaps you are bewildered by the array of titles and pro-grammes defining and describing medical assistants in the USA. Many of you and, indeed, many of us are perplexed and at times concerned by the proliferation of programmes and titles.

Yet, in this seemingly vast array of programmes, efforts, and plans to train and utilize medical assistants, there is a common goal, a desire to improve further the quality and quantity of medical services for all segments of society. It is our sincere belief that such further improvement of medical services will lead to improved health of all our citizens, and this ultimately should lead to improving the quality of life itself, a goal I am confident all nations share.

As varied as the programmes may appear on the surface, there is a common thread in many of them. The majority of those in the USA are directed toward training health personnel capable of providing primary medical care. The desire to improve and increase the availability of primary medical care through the use of medical assistants was a major motivating force in the original develop-ment of these programmes.

It is important to keep in mind that, while the range of primary medical care services that medical assistants provide may be circumscribed and at times prescribed by the training programmes or by legal restrictions, all efforts to train and utilize medical assistants are directed toward improving the quality and quantity of health services. The overall role can best be described as providing primary medical care.

Another point is that the categories or general descriptions under which the medical assistant programmes fall, while varied, in reality can be reduced to two, those that train medical assistants and those that train nurse practitioners. Furthermore, most of these programmes are concerned with curative rather than preventive medicine. I make this last point because in many countries the distinc-tion between curative and preventive medicine is vague, if visible at all. In the USA, on the other hand, the two are quite distinct.

The fundamental question then is: Given that medical assistants and nurse practitioners should be chiefly concerned with primary medical care, and that their services should be directed toward curative medicine, what should be their specific role or roles? In discussing this question, let us confine ourselves to

[1] Bureau of Health Manpower Education, National Institutes of Health, Bethesda, Md.
[2] University of California, San Francisco.

training programmes whether for medical assistants or for nurse practitioners, directed generally toward primary medical care.

EL HAKIM (*Sudan*): The objective of training medical assistants in Sudan is to meet our local health needs and to provide medical services to the sectors of our population living in remote areas. This is slightly different from the assistant physician in the USA. As defined by WHO, the medical assistant is a health worker whose duties include diagnosis and treatment of common diseases. Medical assistants are auxiliaries to a physician and must be under some form of supervision, normally by fully-qualified physicians, or by a senior member of the cadre, such as the senior medical assistant.

Our medical services have a satellite structure beginning with the 30-family dispensary run by what we call the qualified nurse. Five or six of these are linked to a dispensary run solely by a medical assistant. Five or six of the latter units, in turn, constitute a health centre serving approximately 1000 families. Sixty per cent of health centres are run by medical assistants while 40% are run by physicians. At a higher level, the rural hospital serves 5000 families. Medical assistants do not work in the rural hospitals, which are run by physicians as are the next levels in the structure, the district and provincial hospitals. The place of the medical assistant, therefore, is in the dispensary and the health centre.

In addition to his administrative duties, the medical assistant's specific responsibilities are to give first aid in medical and surgical emergencies, to diagnose and treat common ailments and, in the dispensaries, to perform certain approved minor surgical procedures. In addition, he has to carry out special treatments prescribed by the physician, to refer acute and complicated cases to the rural hospital and provide transport for them. In no circumstances may fees be charged for any medical care or medical advice.

In Sudan the medical assistant must carry out all the functions of public health in places where public health officers are not available. He must maintain a close relationship with the local licensed midwife and be available to advise the midwife when complications arise. There should be close liaison and cooperation with the public health authorities, and the medical assistant should be able to detect acute infectious diseases and immediately initiate appropriate sanitary and epidemic control measures. He is also responsible for reporting the occurrence of such cases to the public health medical officer in the area.

In addition, he should be able to carry out health education and answer questions on health from people under his care. As part of his social duties he must educate the population about how to carry out sanitary and health promoting measures He must register all births and deaths, and issue corresponding certificates. He must be able to advise on environmental sanitation, housing, latrines, waste disposal and sewage; he may suspend the sale of any article of food under suspicion until it has been cleared. He advises on nutrition and dietetics, as well as dental care, and he maintains simple administrative records, keeps vital statistics and administers public health laws.

ACUÑA (*Mexico*): In discussing the role of the medical assistant, a survey of the needs that give rise to use of paramedical personnel may be useful.

In Mexico and in many Latin American and Caribbean countries, there is a growing need to extend the coverage of health services. At the present time, the extent and quality of medical assistance are insufficient.

The situation is aggravated by the great discrepancy between the health services provided in rural and in urban areas. In Mexico efforts have been made to widen the activities of the physician in the rural areas, but even if we could produce the required number of qualified medical professionals, the fact is that the economic means to take care of the needs of the extensive rural areas are lacking. Our rural areas are so poor that, generally speaking, communities of 1000 inhabitants cannot economically support a trained physician. I use this figure because it is generally accepted that one physician can attend to 1000 people.

If we consider medical assistants, it is still unrealistic to think in those terms. In other words, we are talking of personnel with basic education who, instead of completing the full curriculum of medical school, internship, and residency, have taken short courses of one, two, or three years. In the final analysis, however, we come back to the same economic problem—at both the professional and the semi-professional level, the individual has to be paid and given the means to work. So perhaps the medical assistant, as defined in these discussions, is not the ideal solution for the rural problems of Latin American and Caribbean countries. We must think of personnel with fewer qualifications and less training.

A possible solution on these lines is now being tried out in Mexico. Selected young people, volunteers, men or women, from small communities of less than 2500 inhabitants, are being trained as auxiliaries to diagnose and treat common diseases. They are given a small medical kit and supply of medicines. The idea is that the community should pay these volunteers, while help is also provided by the Ministry of Health and the health services of the state in which the community is located. This help consists basically of materials for the construction of a small health 'house' (the term 'house' is used to differentiate it from the larger health centre) consisting of two rooms and under the control of a small health committee organized by the community. The person selected for basic training is assigned to the health house and is supervised by a qualified physician from the area health centre who makes visits every four to six weeks. On these visits the physician reviews the records of patients attended, and takes the opportunity to impart further training. Emphasis is placed on referral to the health centre of the more serious cases outside the scope of the volunteer assistant.

Du Gas (*Canada*): There are two reasons why we need a primary health care worker even though we do have very good physician-population and nurse-population ratios. One is the geographical distribution of our population, most of whom live in a narrow 100-mile-wide strip along the American border, with only about 10% inhabiting the vast area of the rest of Canada. We have to deal with numerous small, isolated communities and the consequent transportation problems. We need someone in the physician's assistant category to service these communities.

But we have also found that in the urban areas our primary care services are inadequate. People have difficulty in getting hold of a doctor. The emergency and outpatient departments of our hospitals are overcrowded.

However, we decided that it would be extremely expensive to develop an entirely new category of worker. At a national conference in 1971, when we brought together physicians, nurses, and consumers, it was decided that instead of developing physician's assistants, we would utilize our nurses instead.

One reason for this decision was our very good experience of the use of nurses to provide medical services in northern Canada. Also, we have a large number of nurses, and we thought it better to utilize this resource.

Following the national conference at which this decision was made, a committee was set up to discuss the role and functions of nurse practitioners.

The report of this committee (Boudreau Report) contains a list of functions which the committee thought nurse practitioners would undertake. They are as follows:

'The nurse practitioner can be the initial contact for people entering the health care system, to assess the individual's health status and decide whether referral to a physician is needed.

'The nurse practitioner should be able to initiate treatment for commonly occurring health problems, to do health teaching and health counselling, to look after normal healthy women throughout the maternity cycle, to supervise the health care of well children and the health care of older people, to monitor patients with long-term conditions, to coordinate health care, and to intervene in crisis situations.'

We believe there may be three levels of nurse practitioner: one working in close conjunction with a physician in his practice; one working as a community health nurse, with curative as well as preventive responsibilities; and the more or less independent nurse practitioner who functions as a physician substitute in remote and isolated areas.

In northern communities with populations of 250 persons or more, there is one nurse, for those with over 400 population, there are two. There are a few men nurses, but most are women. The nursing stations are well equipped with radio communication to a base hospital. The doctors make regular visits once a month and specialists come at other times. The nurses can arrange for transport out for patients who need additional services.

However, there is a rapid turnover of staff; most of the nurses do not stay longer than two years, and we must train enough to compensate for the losses.

BEAUSOLEIL (*Ghana*): Three criteria are used in the definition of the medical assistant. These are:

   (a) basic educational standard and level of education;
   (b) duties, responsibilities, and functions;
   (c) duration of training.

The level of education required is bound to vary from country to country and will depend among other things on the most pressing needs to be satisfied and the complexity of the tasks to be performed. It is possible, for instance, to train two people of different educational backgrounds to perform the same tasks with equal competence.

The duration of training is similarly bound to show considerable variation since it will be determined largely by the quality of the people available, the complexity of the tasks, and the degree of competence demanded.

For example, in one country the medical assistant might be required to perform abdominal operations such as appendectomy or caesarean section, while in another country the tasks might be far simpler—the administration of general anaesthesia, diagnosis and treatment of minor ailments, and the referral of cases.

While the training of the former, who is virtually a physician, might take five years, the training of the latter might range from six months to two years.

The duties and responsibilities are also bound to show variation, but it is very easy to specify the duties and responsibilities to be delegated and those that are the prerogative of the physician.

Thus, while a definition based on the educational background or duration of training is likely to lead to misunderstanding and difficulties in acceptance, one based on duties and responsibilities is more likely to be clearly understood and acceptable.

Another matter of concern is the cost of training. One major constraint on the ability of developing countries to develop and expand the health services is an acute shortage of financial resources. In planning any programme, it is important to aim at optimum effectiveness at minimum cost in terms of human, material, and financial resources.

In America, all the programmes are university centred. This is bound to be expensive and unsuitable for a country like mine. Information on the cost of the training programmes would be useful.

RUTASITARA (*Tanzania*): It is clear from what has been said that both the developed and the developing countries represented here have realized the need for a system of health care delivery aimed at (a) ensuring total coverage of the population regardless of social and ethnic differences, and (b) relieving the professional doctor from most of the common and routine activities, thereby allowing him more time to devote to less frequent and often more complex medical problems and time to improve his professional skills. It is in attempting to achieve either or both of these objectives that the need to engage the services of medical auxiliaries arises, even in countries with a standard doctor–patient ratio. Thus, the definition of the medical auxiliary will be determined by the scope of his activity and the role he is given to play.

In the situation prevailing in most developing countries, the chronic lack of professionally qualified medical personnel (i.e., graduate doctors), makes it impossible to man the health services adequately to attain either of the above objectives. However, these countries have undertaken to cover their total populations with some form of medical and health care. Under these circumstances, medical auxiliaries are used to extend the services of the graduate doctors, often at no lower level of quality except in the case of complex medical conditions. However, the medical auxiliaries are not substitutes for the medical doctor. They carry out their duties under the doctor's direct or remote supervision, under his guidance and according to his instructions. The extent to which auxiliaries bear responsibility for their actions while on duty is governed by the circumstances leading to each action. Thus, when they are fully covered by the supervising medical professional, they are not absolutely answerable for their actions. Aptly, some people prefer to call them rural medical practitioners because most of them work in remote rural areas and are rarely visited by qualified doctors. They work more or less independently in their day-to-day activities in dealing with large numbers of simple medical problems and refer the more complicated cases to a far-off, professional doctor. Thus, besides extending the services of the professional doctors, they also filter a large number of medical conditions.

This situation is different from that shown in Dr Smith's film where a medical auxiliary, or medical assistant, is employed to carry out specific medical procedures that will ultimately contribute to the diagnosis and treatment of a particular case by a professionally qualified doctor. Our medical assistants in developing countries do their best, within the limits of their knowledge and experience, to make individual and community diagnoses and initiate treatment and preventive measures without awaiting the opinion of their supervising doctor.

However, we also have medical auxiliaries who assist in carrying out procedures intended to help in the diagnosis or treatment of medical conditions as requested or directed by the doctor. We call them paramedical technical personnel, but they are designated by the type of procedure they undertake. For example, receptionists receive patients and may take the history of the disease, X-ray orderlies take X-rays, and so forth.

In Tanzania medical assistants are employed in the delivery of primary medical and health care at the grass roots in primary health units such as dispensaries, outpatient clinics, and rural health centres. At the intermediate level, there are graduate medical practitioners who are normally in charge of hospitals that serve as referral centres for the primary health units. These doctors are general-duty medical officers who have had a broad medical education at university medical schools. They deal with quite a number of medical and health problems but refer the most complicated ones to higher levels of specialists. The latter have had postgraduate training in broad specialties, such as medicine, surgery, public health, and so forth. A physician, in our case, is a specialist in general medicine.

If, then, a medical assistant trained for the USA programme for the inter-mediate level of health care can be likened to our general medical practitioner, we from developing countries are anxious to see to it that it not only solves the USA problems in the delivery of health care but that it also gives the last blow to the long-standing problem of the brain drain of health manpower by deve-loped countries from the developing ones.

SOOPIKIAN (*Iran*): Developing any new kind of personnel, especially in the medical field, must depend on some overall national policy. If a country decides it wants to have minimum medical coverage for the entire population, then obviously that country cannot depend only on higher professional groups to provide the service: it has to train auxiliaries. Also, if a new type of personnel is introduced, its professional lifespan must be considered. The question should be raised as to how long the group will remain in the overall structure of the country's health services.

Therefore, the first issue to be considered is the general policy of a country governing the use of the medical assistant or any kind of new health personnel. Economic resources, the reaction from the private and public sectors of medicine, and what mixture of private and public health care will provide services must all be taken into account. In Iran the private sector and the public sector are instrumental in providing health services. In the public sector alone, we have 78 different organizations engaged in public health. In introducing a new profes-sion, it is important to determine where it will stand in relation to the entire health care system.

A brief background of Iran's experience in the training of medical assistants may be of interest. Twenty-five years ago we began taking school graduates into a three-year programme to train as medical assistants. After working five years as medical assistants in a rural area, they were permitted to enter the fourth year of the seven-year medical school class. By successfully completing the last three years of medical school, medical assistants became physicians. The programme of training medical assistants was discontinued after ten years largely because many people were referring to them as 'half-baked doctors.' As it turned out they were not really auxiliaries but independent practitioners actually working as physicians in rural areas. Although they were employed by the Government, they were allowed some private practice to supplement their income.

It seemed better to use the physician in our rural areas with a lower auxiliary group. This led to the major decision in Iran to create the health corps team. Physicians who are scheduled for two years of military service can serve the two years in a rural area as part of the health corps. Each physician has two auxiliaries who are high-school graduates with six months' training with a doctor in the rural areas. The health corps teams move from village to village as health needs arise. What is now needed is health personnel who will stay in a village to provide permanent care. At present Iran is considering developing a type of auxiliary who will remain in the villages permanently.

Some further issues that should be considered are those of dependence versus independence, of the general practitioner versus the specialist, of the career span and future of a new or special category of health worker and the time needed for planned services to reach the total population.

When we talk about health care in Iran it must be in relation to a programme developed within a 5-year or a 20-year national programme. We work wth universities and other institutions to try to determine what is the best way to provide health services. It is important also to point out that in Iran the universities are not allowed to initiate a new category of health worker unless it is approved in relation to a total national plan. We want auxiliaries in the rural areas where there are no physicians but where they can still be under the supervision of a physician.

MOUTSOURIS (*Greece*): The state of health manpower in Greece can be outlined in a few words. In a small country like ours with a population of 8 000 000, there are some 12 000 or 12 500 physicians, which provides a ratio of one physician to approximately 600 people.

By law, upon completion of his university training, every physician is obliged to practise in a rural area for one year. This is obligatory and no exceptions are made. No hospital or university will accept a physician for further training unless he has fulfilled that obligation.

The country has been divided into a number of defined rural areas to which all doctors go. In small towns of 5000 population, the physician is assisted by a midwife and a nurse.

The term of medical assistant is unknown in Greece. There are no schools or written programmes for medical assistants, but Greece does have programmes for midwives, physical therapists, public health technicians, and supervisors of hospital administration. There has been talk of developing a programme which would call for training in a health field at an educational level between high school and university. But in no sense can this be called a programme for training medical assistants.

While Greece does not have a shortage of physicians, it has a problem of unequal distribution of medical manpower. This problem of maldistribution, however, is being solved by the Government through the requirement that each physician practise in a rural area for one year.

DIESH (*India*): Taking into account the population structure, the morbidity pattern, and the problems of illiteracy, ignorance, and poverty, our main endeavour in India is to integrate not only preventive and curative medicine but also family planning into a system of total health care. Our objective is to provide minimum medical coverage to the maximum number of people in a minimum period.

We have developed an extensive network of health services in the rural areas in the form of primary health centres. But due to lack of sufficient numbers of trained health personnel, these services are still very fragile.

Despite large-scale efforts to train doctors, maldistribution of doctors within the country continues. It is estimated that 80% of the doctors settle in urban areas, leaving only 20% of the available physicians to serve the 82% of our population who live in rural areas and who contribute 70% of our national economy.

The aim of training and making effective use of all members of the health team offers the greatest challenge in the health field today. A method of health care delivery must be developed and expanded in order to bring better care to the largest number of people in the community. Thus has arisen the urgent need to develop a medical team with paramedical workers to provide integrated and comprehensive health services.

It is understood that the greatest returns will come from increased investment in the intermediate level of health workers. Relevant training and effective use of paramedical workers are fundamental if health services are to be improved and the cost of medical care reduced.

In the present context of development of health services in the country, it is more desirable to overproduce personnel in the paramedical category who do not have an exportable university qualification than, at great expense, to overproduce physicians who are exportable.

We have various categories of medical aids such as nurses, health assistants, sanitary inspectors, auxiliary nurse midwives, health visitors, public health nurses, basic health workers, and so forth. These medical assistants have a major role to play in different parts of the country, particularly in the remote areas where the doctors do not go. We are trying to develop this category of health worker with proper training for service to the community.

TADELLE (*Ethiopia*): I have three brief comments. The first relates to the role of the medical assistant, which ought to be determined on the basis of the socio-economic condition of a country. Furthermore, the historical context in which the training of medical assistants has developed should be given due attention.

Second, the need for medical assistants should not be judged on the basis of single factors such as reduced cost of training, shortage of doctors, or the need to ease unemployment. On the other hand, in defining the need for medical assistants and their role, the health care system should be considered in its totality.

Third, we should distinguish between medical assistants trained primarily to increase the efficiency of physicians and those who are trained mainly to provide basic health services.

DIEN (*Viet-Nam*): In Viet-Nam we make a distinction between medical personnel and auxiliary health personnel. There is a great shortage of physicians. With approximately one physician per 2000 population, we believe programmes to train auxiliary health personnel must be developed.

In addition to doctors of medicine, we have people called auxiliary physicians. These are workers who obtained four years of instruction at the University of Hanoi. Most of them are old and retired, but some continue to practise.

At another level we have 'medical assistants', who are low level workers and not comparable with the medical assistants in a number of other countries as described during this conference.

Health workers in the military category may be classified as nurses, technicians, and health officers. In the civilian category there are public health workers, midwives, physiotherapists, X-ray technicians, and the like. These are usually referred to as health auxiliaries and function either as aids or as technicians.

A further distinction is that individuals classified as 'health technicians' have three years of training, whereas those classified as 'health auxiliaries' have only a primary certificate.

Another category of health worker in Viet-Nam is the private or irregular nurse; there are approximately 23 000 of them. These irregular nurses are legally allowed to give almost any treatments, including those usually performed by physicians.

It is important again to emphasize that the term 'medical assistant' in Viet-Nam leads to confusion because there are several categories of individuals who come under this title. In Viet-Nam, as in almost all other developing countries, we use a health worker comparable to the medical assistant, an individual who is competent to perform medical services.

SILVER (*USA*): It seems that a problem in communication exists. We have used a variety of terms for the 'medical assistant.' These have included such terms as physician's assistant, MEDEX, physician associate, and many others.

I believe it would be reasonable for us to adopt a single term for this entire group of health workers. It might not be generally adopted by the public but used primarily by us. The word I am suggesting is 'syniatrist'; its Greek derivations means 'with' ('syn') and 'physician' ('iatrist'). I am suggesting that this term be used to designate those health workers below the level of the medical doctor. 'Syniatrist' could be modified according to the level of competence of an individual.

The highest level, the 'syniatrist associate' would be the individual capable of relatively autonomous action. He need not actually be independent, but he would be capable of doing many things on his own. He could be someone who is now called a physician's assistant in the USA. Or it could be a nurse or a medical assistant. This person would be capable of independent action, of making decisions, and taking action on his own.

The second level of syniatrist would be the 'syniatrist assistant.' He would be someone capable of serving as a well-trained medical technician and of performing a variety of duties and functions, but only because he had been trained to do so. He would not be expected to serve in an autonomous or independent fashion. His actions would be based on specific guidelines and standing orders.

The third type of syniatrist would be the 'syniatrist aid.' This would be an individual who had received essentially no formal training, and he would limit himself to rather routine types of activities.

If we used a classification of this kind, our ability to communicate with others would be improved when it came to describing and discussing various types of 'medical assistants.' The classification would apply to health workers in all countries.

ROSINSKI (*USA*): I would probably disagree with Dr Silver because I really do not think that the name is the point at issue. The issue is one of differences of opinion about the concept of the role of the medical assistant.

The training and utilization of medical assistants are subjects to which all of you have made extremely significant contributions this morning. The USA has followed your leadership in many of the areas which you have described in the training and utilization of medical assistants. It was a concept alien to most of us some 10 or 12 years ago, and in numerous cases we have benefited from your experience.

From the various programmes you have described, the responsibilities of medical assistants in reality are not too different. There is a thread of similarity in what all of us are trying to do—provide some form of primary medical care of good quality. As has been pointed out, the specific role of the medical assistant will depend considerably on the social and economic background of the country, as well as the country's overall health objectives. Furthermore, since all of us are striving to increase the quantity and improve the quality of health care for all our citizens, the use of the medical assistant appears as one way to achieve that highly desirable goal.

Another significant point repeatedly made is that the reason for developing medical assistants is not to relieve the physician of his or her professional responsibilities. On the contrary, it is to have the medical assistant serve as an assistant to the physician so that the physician may extend his or her professional services to a large segment of the population. This is a crucial point that must be considered as nations seek to develop medical assistant programmes.

The concern about the proliferation of programmes is extremely important. All of us are faced with the problem of how to regulate the development and proliferation of programmes, especially since some seem to be growing haphazardly.

And finally, the caution lest the role of the medical assistant should become too similar to that of the physician is of particular importance. As the distinction between the physician and the medical assistant becomes less clear-cut, we may run into a considerable amount of difficulty, not only with society in general, but with our professional colleagues. The distinction between the MD and the medical assistant must always be kept to the forefront as we develop training programmes and utilize medical assistants.

———

TRAINING

Chairman: *THOMAS HATCH*[1]
Moderator: *DOUGLAS FENDERSON, Ph.D.*[1]

FENDERSON (*USA*): Our subject is training. What shall we teach, to whom, to what end, and how?

The first issue regarding training is the relationship of the training programme to the system or the setting within which the workers will function. In the USA we do not have a single system, in a formal sense, for the delivery of health care. We tend, therefore, to have many kinds of programmes to meet differently perceived needs and problems.

The second issue is the purpose of the training. Is the purpose mainly to give more individual opportunity to students, or is it to meet the needs of a health care system? For example, there is an extremely large number of applicants for the 40 available places in the Duke University physician's assistant programme, because this role is seen as personally advantageous. And while self-interest is appropriate, many of your remarks indicate an overriding concern for the solution of public problems.

The basis for development of the curriculum is an important issue. Fendall[2] says that every country, every setting, every particular environment within which these people are to be employed must be subjected to some kind of market and task analysis and that curricula should be developed on the basis of such studies rather than as a result of the competing pressures of different groups. But how do we determine what knowledge and skills are required? Is there some objective basis for specifying the objectives of training programmes?

With respect to subject matter, Dr Estes indicated earlier that educators, in consultation with practising physicians, had designed a programme which has been refined on the basis of experience and study. Dr Smith indicated that an analysis of tasks and the special characteristics of a particular medical practice setting were used to define a particular student's preparation. That is contrary to an earlier suggestion that standardization of the role, at least within a given country, is essential. Fendall studied the frequency distribution of medical problems seen in dispensing clinics in a number of developing countries. On the basis of his appraisal of the medical skills and knowledge required, he concluded that 90% of the medical conditions seen could be treated by intermediate level personnel, between 5% and 10% required more formal medical treatment and between 2% and 5% required hospitalization. Fendall also suggested the use of epidemiological surveys in local areas.

[1] Bureau of Health Manpower Education, National Institutes of Health, Bethesda, Md.
[2] Fendall, N. R. E. (1972) *Auxiliaries in health care; programs in developing countries*, Baltimore & London, Johns Hopkins Press (Josiah Macy Foundation).

Is the purpose of the curriculum to train to specified levels of technical competence or to provide a broad educational background to which technical skills are added? There is some criticism in the USA of the tendency to produce narrowly defined technicians who ultimately have dead-end jobs, unsatisfying careers, and limited occupational tenure. It has been suggested that workers, if trained in such a limited way, could be exploited by professional and managerial groups and made to do jobs that are not particularly desirable or profitable for other groups.

Should the training be a shadow of medical education or should it be an entirely new kind of training, based on some organizing principle, such as the function-oriented curriculum described by Dr Smith?

Fendall's study recommends that training be one-third didactic and two-thirds clinical, carried out largely in an apprenticeship in a clinical setting. He says greater efficiency can be obtained if the training takes place in what we would call an academic health science centre, though he cautions against fragmenting the curriculum. He believes that training should be pragmatic rather than scientific. The number of instructors, therefore, should be limited, and all material not essential to the defined functions should be excluded.

We know that apprenticeship training works well. It is a time-honoured method, certainly, in the training of physicians, for whom clinical training is essential. But we also know that academic training has great influence and efficiency. The question then centres on the mix of formal academic programmes and clinical apprenticeships that can lead effectively and efficiently to the desired outcome.

Who shall be selected? There is a tendency for training programmes for auxiliaries to raise entry standards and to lengthen courses to a greater extent than is actually required to fit trainees for the job; this leads to 'overqualification of applicants.' Perhaps there is a need for more discussion on the point.

NATHANIELS (*Togo*): It is undeniable that a scarcity of qualified medical personnel exists throughout the world. Each country must develop its programme and system of instruction according to the means it possesses, and, above all, according to its needs for qualified medical personnel.

In the light of earlier discussions, it is evident that in Togo we are seeking a different goal from that of the programmes in the United States. Nevertheless, we will take as a model the system of training in foreign universities while adapting it to the problems of the health infrastructure in our country.

I was impressed by the report of Dr Estes regarding his ten-year experience in the training of medical assistants at Duke University as well as by the bold programme for training medical assistant specialists at the University of Colorado.

With several variations, our programme approaches that of the School of Medical Assistants at Duke University. Their programme is concerned principally with curative medicine, while we give priority to preventive medicine and public health. Instruction is intended for nurses, midwives, laboratory assistants and sanitation personnel who can show evidence of a minimum of five years of practice as a full-time member of a health team. The school fixes the lower and upper age limits at 24 years and 40 years.

Recruitment is by way of a competitive examination. Last year we accepted only 27 candidates out of the 169 who took this entrance examination.

Teaching is multidisciplinary and consists of three distinct sections which correspond to the previous professional activities of the student: medical studies; studies in sanitary engineering; and studies in advanced laboratory techniques.

The medical studies leading to the university degree of medical assistant are concise, concrete, and accelerated. They include basic training in human sciences, demography, law, etc. and theoretical training in basic medical sciences, general and specialty medicine, tropical medicine, surgery and surgical specialties, obstetrics and gynaecology, preventive medicine, public health organization and pedagogy.

From the first year, students function as hospital students in the University Hospital Centre of Lomé, taking patients' histories, and assisting in consultations. In the spring term, they are assigned for two-week periods in the health centres in rural areas. For two months in the summer, they assist physicians in regional hospital centres.

Following recommendations of the World Health Organization and the minimal standards fixed by that organization for the training and equivalence of diplomas as medical laboratory technicians, students at the medical laboratories of our school will obtain the diploma given by the University of Benin when they have successfully followed a two-year programme of study including both theory and practice, with emphasis on the latter.

Our school also trains sanitary engineering technicians. This section is open to former sanitarians admitted by examination to the school. The programme approximates to that of the Centre of Sanitary Engineering at the University of Rabat.

Emphasis has been placed principally on the basic elements of public health (communicable diseases, bacteriology, sanitation, demographic statistics, etc.). Courses are given on the techniques of construction, technology of concrete, hydro-electric installations, hydraulic engineering and fluid mechanics, road construction, soil mechanics, hydrology, and sanitary engineering. The courses in sanitary engineering have been organized in cooperation with the World Health Organization. This training is intended to prepare sanitary engineering technicians to work in a team with doctors.

MINKOLA-NDOSIMA (*Zaire*): The Republic of Zaire has had different types of medical assistants for a long time. Before 1960 all medical personnel were trained in the school of medicine. The nurse, the medical assistant, and all medical personnel were trained with the same orientation and in the same elements of diagnostics and treatment.

The medical assistant was an assistant to the doctor. He could be found either in the hospital or in distant parts of the country. He was responsible for taking the medical history, for carrying out the preliminary examination, and for giving the treatment prescribed.

In the rural areas, the medical assistant was always under the legal responsibility of a supervising physician. Although physically far away, he carries out the same type of functions as the physician. He sent cases that were too difficult for him to the nearest hospital.

When the medical assistant job was established in 1936, the training was among the most advanced in the country. The medical assistant started his studies at the end of secondary school. His training lasted four years with an additional two years of internship, which was also a kind of probationary period. He had successfully to complete the two years of internship under the direction of a doctor, and his work had to be approved by the supervising physician.

103

In 1960, when the country became independent, we created another category —graduates in medicine. This category emerged as part of the general revision of training programmes in the country and was of a higher level than that of the medical assistant. Because our country did not have any MDs, graduates in medicine wanted sooner or later to become doctors of medicine, and the political authorities had certain problems at the social level. For a time the training was considered unsuitable because we spent a lot of money to train a graduate in medicine who would not remain in that role. For that reason the programme was suspended temporarily.

WATSON (*Papua New Guinea*): The middle-level worker is not a doctor. He should be trained for his special role from the first day of his training. When a doctor sees a patient who says he has a cough, the doctor thinks of a list of possible causes for that cough.

An immediate short cut in the training of the less sophisticated worker is to teach him a symptom differential process for making a specific diagnosis or a sort of group diagnosis. An example of the latter is anaemia, which in Papua New Guinea is commonly caused either by malaria, or by dietary deficiency, or by hookworm. Because he is not trained to use the microscope, pathology tests, or X-rays, our health extension officer is not taught to seek beyond 'anaemia', although he must be aware of the possible causes. He is taught a standard regime for managing anaemia. This is disgraceful 'shotgun therapy' in a developed country, but for this man it is good management.

He needs a standard drug regime rather than a variety of regimes. Doctors can consult a number of different textbooks. They are encouraged to select wisely from many possible alternatives. There is no room for this kind of luxury in the training of our auxiliaries.

The man needs to be trained for his definitive role. He needs to feel pride in it from the time he starts his training until he retires. He should not see it as a stopping place on the way to somewhere else. A doctor who works for a year in a rural area, or a doctor who does a couple of years in military service, is obviously just 'marking time.' The auxiliary must see his work as a career.

He needs his own textbooks. Perhaps in developed countries he does not need them so much; he is already a highly educated man. We print health extension officer texts, and are developing others which are as yet only duplicated.

Our man is indeed an intermediate-level worker; we have another worker below him. So an important part of the health extension officer's role is to supervise the workers below him and to delegate some of this responsibilities to them.

This kind of training has been described as pragmatic rather than scientific. It is scientific, however, in that you determine what health care is needed and feasible, and then develop a method of training to meet that need.

DIEN (*Viet-Nam*): Under the French influence in Viet-Nam, a kind of super-nurse or medical assistant course was created in 1942. That course was interrupted in 1945 because of political events, and students finished their last year of study in 1949.

My comments concern the study programmes for these medical assistants. They had to pass written examinations and a physical endurance test, part of which was to bicycle 10 kilometres. I question whether this physical aptitude test is really necessary in the competition for admission of health technicians.

Another comment concerns the admissions into the nursing service under the Health Ministry in my country. In addition to subjects that have been mentioned by our colleagues, we have a three-month vocational observation period following which the candidates begin special nursing studies. I am not sure that the observation period is necessary any longer, since the nursing student, after three years of studies, has already had a vocational observation period.

We have a problem in the curriculum for the irregular nurses, who are particularly respected persons. They take special evening courses of one to two hours duration for only three to four months. They have a different and quite traditional kind of training which does not always conform to the theory and practice which we teach.

FERNANDO (*Ceylon*): You have quite rightly organized the discussion to include both the roles and the training; these cannot be divorced. Training often proceeds without consideration of the trainee's role.

We have different categories of workers. In the past, each was trained separately and worked in isolation. Now, however, there is the team concept in health. Having accepted that, we should not train people for certain jobs without examining the entire curriculum. If the team concept is accepted, the curriculum should reflect the team approach. Our response to the questions the moderator put to us is that we believe it is time to examine training in its entirety. If we are to develop the team concept, we must redistribute our curriculum within the various groups.

I agree with the moderator that there is too much talk about pragmatism and scientific medicine. There is also talk about the science and art of medicine. We think that we are scientific and that we are learning science, and we have forgotten the art of medicine. Why can we not accept that pragmatism can be taught in a scientific way and yet is not science? The curriculum should be more task-oriented and job-oriented, particularly for the medical assistant. In working out *what* and *to what end*, we should not again disassociate the medical assistant from the other workers, especially the doctor.

We must avoid ill-defined roles and merging curricula, otherwise we will end up in a chaotic situation.

FILHO (*Brazil*): In Brazil there is a great deal of regional variation with respect to needs, resources, and development. In Paraiba we have both physicians and auxiliary personnel. We have a health plan which requires us to assess our health care deficiencies, such as the lack of health coverage for 33 % of the population— principally a lack of mother and child care. Thus, what is of particular concern for us is the training of midwives.

We do not have the kind of medical assistant discussed in this meeting. As Dr Acuña mentioned, Brazil and Mexico have similar problems. We are more concerned about personnel at the lowest levels, people who can provide care to the rural populations.

TABIBZADEH (*Iran*): When we started our medical assistants programme 26 or 27 years ago, perhaps we did not give too much consideration to the importance of the level of training. We recruited high-school graduates and gave them four complete years of training, almost exactly the same as is given in the medical school. After five or six years, these people got together and formed a small association and asked to enter the fourth year of the medical school. This was refused.

The training of the medical assistant depends on a clear definition of objectives and needs. It must also recognize the purposes for which they are being trained and who should train them. Our experience has shown that training by a very scientific academic group is not practical for the type of medical assistant we have been training.

TADELLE (*Ethiopia*): The essential questions have been raised by Dr Fenderson. However, I would like to make some observations about the training of medical assistants.

The first involves the separation between preventive and curative medicine. It is not unusual to hear that one is more important than the other, but it should be noted that such an emphasis, if it exists, should not be taken into consideration in measuring the success or failure of a training scheme.

The evaluation of a training programme is an important and necessary task, but it has not been given the priority it deserves in terms of staff and time required for the purpose. Furthermore, evaluation should be undertaken as far as possible by the nationals of a country with the assistance of WHO and other agencies.

The training of medical assistants and of the physicians who are supposed to supervise them should be compatible. It is likely that medical schools in developing countries are or will become carbon copies of their counterparts in Europe and North America. In comparison, schools for medical assistants are new and are designed to solve local problems and needs. Attempts should be made to correct training incompatibilities.

The question of recruiting able teachers for medical assistants as well as that of the feedback of information from the graduates to the schools where the training is given are still in suspense. I would like to hear more on these issues from my colleagues.

RUTASITARA (*Tanzania*): My intention is to describe the categories of people in my country that go by the name of 'medical assistant.'

A physician in my country is a specialist in general medicine, and his cases are referred to him by a general medical practitioner, who is also a medical graduate. Therefore, the term 'physician's assistant' would not apply in my country. It is below the level of the general medical practitioner that we have several categories of medical assistants.

First, at the grass roots in the village, there is a first-aider or village medical helper. This is a person trusted by members of the village to arrange for their medical and health care. Often, but not necessarily, he is a primary-school leaver without medical training other than first-aid experience acquired either in a hospital or in an organization such as the Red Cross. He does not practise medicine but can be trusted to carry out instructions left by medical or health teams. For example, in the control of communicable diseases such as tuberculosis and leprosy, he can be trusted with the drugs to be dispensed to patients in prescribed doses and intervals.

Above the village medical helper, we have a rural medical aid. This is a primary-school leaver who has undergone a three-year training period in curative and preventive medicine. He is usually a leader of the health team at a dispensary that serves approximately 10 000 people. He makes diagnoses and initiates treatment and preventive measures in his area. He refers the difficult cases to the medical assistant or even to doctors at higher levels. However, he is frequently supervised by the doctor or the medical assistant.

The medical assistant proper is usually in charge of a rural health centre that ideally serves five satellite dispensaries in an area with about 50 000 people. Cases are referred to him from the satellite dispensaries. He supervises all health workers in his area and he implements health plans as directed by his superior officer, the district medical officer.

106

Candidates for training as medical assistants should have completed four years of secondary education with good performance in science subjects. Candidates may also be exceptionally good rural medical aids who have worked in that grade for not less than three years. They undergo a three-year training course in curative and preventive medicine, in addition to basic biomedical subjects related to their clinical practice. Up to this level nobody is allowed to undertake surgery other than dressing superficial wounds and incising superficial abscesses. They are also not allowed to use more than prescribed simple medicaments in the treatment of diseases. They cannot practise midwifery and gynaecology.

As already mentioned, the medical assistant is ever craving to get nearer the grade of the doctor, if not to become one. We have tried to bring their knowledge closer to the professional level by arranging an 18 months upgrading course. This is an apprenticeship course in the major disciplines of medicine, including basic lectures in biomedical sciences. Those that successfully complete the course can become licensed medical practitioners in central government, state or voluntary agency health organizations. They are not allowed to set up private practice, and their license expires once they leave the services of these organizations. They are equivalent to the MEDEX of the programme at the University of Washington. The only difference is that our assistant medical officers, as they are called, can substitute for doctors rather than extend their services. They are loosely addressed as doctors.

A few of these assistant medical officers, however, have now been selected to join the University for the MD course along with other medical students.

DIESH (*India*): In India we have attempted to develop rural health services through a 'minimum need programme.' In fact, India's Fifth Five Year Plan is entirely for the rural health services with practically nothing for the urban areas. In the execution of this programme our endeavour is to utilize the different kinds of paramedical and health assistants who are available in the country. For each category of workers, we have laid down the job description, the curriculum content, training needs, duration of the course, and so forth. We have also ascertained the facilities that are available and estimated the additional facilities that will be needed during the Fifth Five Year Plan.

In this connexion, WHO is helping to organize the training programmes of these paramedical and health assistants. Under the programme, there will be six national centres in the country for which WHO and UNICEF will provide assistance in reorienting existing health assistants and medical auxiliaries, as well as in training the teachers.

BEAUSOLEIL (*Ghana*): Like the roles and functions of the medical assistant, training programmes are bound to vary from country to country and one cannot offer any hard and fast rules. All that can be attempted is to offer guidelines embracing certain fundamental principles that may be summarized as follows:

1. A detailed task description should be drawn up.

2. The objectives of a training programme should be formulated on the basis of the task description.

3. The syllabus and curriculum should be developed on the basis of the training objectives.

4. A special cadre of teachers and instructors for auxiliary health workers should be established.

5. In deciding upon the minimum entry qualifications of candidates, a special effort must be made to avoid specifying the same qualifications as those

required for the professional grade; good incentives and a career structure are also necessary in order to avoid frustration and loss to professional schools.

The validity of these principles is obvious, but it is sad to observe that they are often overlooked, with disastrous results.

In Ghana we have found it advantageous to use and apply modern educational technology in training programmes and are seeking assistance from WHO in this connexion.

ACUÑA (*Mexico*): It is interesting to note that, on the one hand, most of the contributions during the previous session were made by professors representing distinguished universities in the USA, and, on the other, that the experiences that have just been described in relation to the training of auxiliary or paramedical personnel referred to courses organized by the ministries or departments of health in developing countries. It would appear then that in Latin America and certain countries of Africa, Asia, and the Middle East, this responsibility is outside the sphere of the universities. Generally, the public health schools are not affiliated with universities but depend on the ministries of health. In this connexion (and I refer specifically to my own country) the universities are criticized for not being up-to-date insofar as their programmes do not meet the real needs of the country. They produce, traditionally, the professionals that they, the universities, consider to be needed. Thus, if the universities do not turn out the type of professional required from a social and economic stand-point, the ministries have necessarily to take over that responsibility, and establish schools of public health and special courses to train auxiliary and paramedical personnel. This, I suggest, is a great waste of time, effort, and resources. The experience, costly installations, equipment, and facilities of the universities could well be taken advantage of to produce not only qualified physicians but also the type of paramedical personnel and auxiliaries required by the country. In suggesting this, I am not losing sight of the insistence of the universities on certain academic requirements, but the fact is that their reluctance to reduce the level of those requirements has resulted in a separation between them and those responsible for providing the health services. It would be a source of congratulation if these differences could be resolved in the true interest of the country.

EL HAKIM (*Sudan*): The training of medical assistants started in the Sudan in 1918 shortly after the first World War. The original programme was one of undertraining which gradually progressed to our modern system of selecting and training the best candidates. The conditions the candidate should fulfil for enrolment in the Medical Assistants Training School at Omdurman Hospital are well defined. He must have successfully completed the nine years of basic education, he must have obtained the nursing certificate which is granted after completion of three years' training, and he should have done three years' work in a hospital, health centre, or dispensary after getting his nursing certificate, i.e., to have spent a total of six or seven years' working as a nurse. Candidates from all the provinces of the Sudan who have fulfilled these conditions are required to take the competitive examination held by the School; those who obtain the highest marks are enrolled. The number of candidates ranges from 100 to 120, with an average enrolment ranging from 43 to 45.

The course of training takes two years and really should be extended to three years because special subjects such as paediatrics, mental diseases, forensic medicine, industrial and school health have been added to the curriculum. Students are not finding the time for their clinical and practical training.

The curriculum consists of 2032 hours, of which 640 hours are for theoretical studies and 1392 hours for practical and clinical work. All teaching is done by physicians. At the conclusion of training, all candidates take a national examination.

The whole training programme is the responsibility of three full-time doctors of the Ministry of Health, one of whom is the principal of the school.

I want to emphasize that in the Sudan it is a single, unified programme designed to avoid complications and confusion. Though the term 'medical assistant' is perhaps not a good one, we consider it the best choice because these are the same type of people, with the same conditions of work and with the same role in the medical field.

I was very much impressed with Dr Smith's discussion of the physician's assistant. He said that in his MEDEX programme he had selected some of the nursing staff, but he did not indicate if they would become physician's assistants or if they would be qualified for another role.

SMITH (*USA*): Let me answer Dr Hakim's question by saying that we were invited by the Government of Micronesia to develop a MEDEX programme in which they adopted our guidelines to train an intermediate cadre. They requested that we start with a group of nurses and health assistants simultaneously, and we began training them simultaneously in the same class.

They took their best potential providers of primary care (nurses), and during the next year or so will continue to produce a decreasing number of graduate nurses and more health assistants. In this way, they will develop a fairly high level of health care provider for this vast area of Micronesia. But the idea is not to take away from nursing because nurses are needed very badly. It was simply that in the first few classes they wanted to get the best possible people available.

These people are in an age group that will not have the ambition to go on to the medical school. This was another reason for their selection.

DY (*WHO Regional Director, Manila*): When I learned about the convening of this conference from Dr Flahault last January, I immediately informed him that I should like to come and attend it as an observer.

The reason is that in the Western Pacific Region, it is extremely urgent and important to use so-called medical assistants if we are going to do something about the terrific lack of delivery of health and medical services, particularly in the rural areas. Most of the countries in the Region, except Australia, Japan and New Zealand, are developing. In these countries, where 70% to 80% of the people live in the rural areas and where up to 70% die without medical attention, the situation is grave. We must do something; governments must do something. That is the reason why this conference is timely and important.

If I may speak frankly, at least for the Western Pacific Region, the use and training of physician's assistants, in the context of the USA's experience, is probably considered not as urgent and not as important at this time as the training and utilization of the medical assistants of a lower level. We have heard that the physician's assistants programme in the USA is progressing quite well. However, it is more oriented to curative medicine. This is, of course, logical in view of the socioeconomic development of the country.

In the developing countries of the Western Pacific Region, however, the needs are simpler and include the establishment of basic health services and the extension of the benefits of medical progress to the poor people in the rural areas. Emphasis should be given more to preventive medicine, including maternal and child health, basic sanitation, immunization, health statistics, and so on.

Dr Diesh mentioned, the emphasis should be more on rural health work rather than on urban health services.

This is the reason why most participants, in discussing this subject, could not help mentioning the problems which involve the training and utilization of the lower level of medical assistants.

Perhaps the Fogarty International Center might consider convening another conference with emphasis on the medical assistants of a less sophisticated type or of a lower level. Because this is an important problem, we in the Western Pacific Region are convening a seminar on the subject, probably lasting ten days, in 1975.

HATCH (*USA*): Thank you, Dr Dy. There are many people, even in the USA, who would echo your words about the need for more attention to preventive medicine. Our moderator, Dr Fenderson, will summarize this discussion.

FENDERSON (*USA*): Several themes were emphasized in this discussion:

1. The level of the educational programme is based on the systems of education and health care in a given country.

2. Training should be based on a careful definition of the role and functions to be performed and in relation to the various other types of health workers.

3. Training is based on a different principle than training of physicians. It is task and technique oriented, and although its scientific content may be less than that required in training physicians, the approach should be no less careful and well thought out. There is a danger of training at too high a level, and this could create role conflict and dissatisfaction.

4. Selection of people who are likely to remain in the areas of greatest need should be considered. The principle is that of local recruitment for local service.

5. A specific recommendation was made for the evaluation of training programmes, perhaps with the consultative assistance of an international group such as WHO, and as part of that evaluation, consideration should be given to the personal experience of the medical auxiliaries.

6. The availability of teachers is a matter of concern; training of teachers needs to be considered.

And finally, there is a role for WHO to assist in the training of teachers, in helping to define the curriculum, and in providing some consultative assistance with regard to the evaluation of training programmes.

CAREER STATUS

Chairman: VICTOR W. SIDEL, M.D.[1]

Moderator: RICHARD A. SMITH, M.D.[2]

SIDEL (*USA*): I was fortunate to be able to make some studies in 1967 on the role and training of the feldsher in the Soviet Union, and in 1971 and 1972 on the role and training of the barefoot doctor in the People's Republic of China.

The 'feldsher model,' that of a technology-based assistant, has been very adequately presented by earlier speakers. The 'barefoot doctor model,' a very different one which might be termed 'community-based' rather than 'technology-based,' has not often been mentioned in this conference, probably because its subject is 'Intermediate levels of health care personnel.' I would like to join Dr Dy and the others who spoke earlier in urging that at a future conference models for the medical assistant like the barefoot doctor be presented and discussed. These models might emphasize community participation and motivation rather than technical skills.

SMITH (*USA*): A discussion of the development of the career status of medical assistants can be approached in two ways. One point of view is that here is an opportunity to train individuals for a professionally stimulating and satisfying career in a specific category for which scarce human and financial resources have been allocated. Another is that here is an opportunity to provide a career ladder to accommodate the medical assistant's inherent desire for promotion.

Important also is the matter of professional identity and self-image, and of the image perceived by the public. If a medical assistant is ashamed of his identity and does not have a clear image of himself, he cannot expect others to have confidence in his image.

Therefore, it is important to emphasize the development of clear and precise identities for medical assistants, identities that are comforting to patients as well as to professional colleagues. Otherwise, these individuals will attempt to portray themselves as something they are not or try to move out of their category.

Dr Rex Fendall of Liverpool, whose writing in this field is familiar to many of you, recently visited two of our MEDEX programmes here in the USA. After spending two hours alone with two experienced MEDEX, he emerged impressed by their competence and commitment. He expressed surprise, moreover, that they had good images of themselves in a professionally satisfying career. He wondered why he had spent two hours trying to persuade them to go to medical school. They were where they wanted to be and they were satisfied with their career status.

[1] Montefiore Hospital, Bronx, New York.
[2] University of Hawaii School of Medicine, Honolulu, Hawaii.

111

However, many of us, Dr Fendall included, believe that maximum career mobility should be provided for categories such as medical assistants. I mention this example because I believe that, if attention is given to this important matter, solutions to the problem of career status can be found.

One can ask why training for this new cadre cannot be used as a stepping stone to other careers? If individuals do not have the initial requirements to enter a higher level of job, then this type of training may provide them with the only opportunity to upgrade themselves. Although it is socially and economically expensive, some degree of mobility must be allowed to individuals within the large domain of health professions. But perhaps it would be wise to limit it to the most promising candidates.

SOOPIKIAN (*Iran*): Dr Todd mentioned earlier that in the USA there are 18 programmes varying from eight weeks to five years, and that the institutions offering this type of training are in the private sector, in colleges, in medical institutions, and universities. The types of degree obtainable may be master's degree, bachelor's degree, certificate, or nothing at all.

In Iran, we have come to the conclusion that this type of career should be limited to the public sector: medical auxiliaries should be trained and used in the health system in the public sector and should not be allowed private practice. Our private sector is assuming a greater responsibility in the hospitals and in providing specialized care.

In our country, we specially want to send this group to the rural areas to work as employees in the national health service. They should have the opportunty to progress up the service ladder, to move to better geographical locations, and to obtain additional training.

The career depends upon the type of training. If we train these people to a master's degree level, it is a quite different type of profession—what I call the half-baked doctor. What is needed is a real auxiliary group primarily for the remote areas and to help doctors in some situations in the cities. Programmes should be designed to keep them in their career rather than to encourage them to become medical doctors, though some very promising ones may do so. Their work should be limited to the public sector.

It is important that this group should be able to see where they stand in the total health structure so that even 20 years later they will know where they fit in that picture. They should not think of themselves as people meeting a temporary need who will later be forgotten. Their image of their career and the satisfactions they gain from that career are very important.

NATHANIELS (*Togo*): Problems created by the lack of qualified health personnel and the need for socioeconomic development are real issues in Togo.

In the general framework of the civil service in Togo, officers are classed in two main categories: top civil servants and civil servants belonging to a middle category. However, the government offers the possibility for promotion to members of the middle category. The latter can gain access to the upper cadre by way of complementary training in their respective branches, obtained either in our national institutions or overseas.

Nurses showing particular promise are given an opportunity for promotion, through courses either at our university or by correspondence.

We have five cadres within the two main categories:

First category

Cadre A-1: The top of the scale with at least a doctorate degree.

Cadre A-2: Licenciate or equivalent.

Second category

Cadre B: The level of the baccalaureate (12 years basic training) or equivalent technical training.

Cadre C: B.E.P.C. (9 years basic training) with at least 2 years of technical training.

Cadre D: Primary school certificate with technical training varying from six months to one year.

The problem of paramedical personnel presents itself in three ways:

1. There is a lack of intermediate level health personnel that we have tried to meet by creating a school of medical assistants under the auspices of the University of Benin at Lomé.

2. The opportunity for career promotion offered to medical assistants.

3. Attempts to stop the loss of valuable workers from the public health services.

The student who has finished his three years of training obtains a university degree which is the equivalent of a licence. He can then be integrated into cadre A-2 of the Togolese civil service. Medical assistants who have worked as paramedical workers in our hospitals and who have carried out periods of specialization as, for example, in ophthalmology, in anaesthesia, in diagnostic X-ray, in dental surgery, can, at the end of their studies, be assigned as medical assistant specialists in hospitals where there is a lack of such specialists.

HARDIN (*Malaysia*): Historically, my country has been making use of this type of medical assistant for about 25 years. They are called hospital assistants. They receive the same training as nurses, plus an additional six to nine months of training in diagnosis and treatment.

In spite of tremendous progress in recent years, we shall be needing this grade of personnel for a long time to come, not only to man the many remote facilities in our country but also to assist doctors in the daily routine work in the hospital.

To provide a career structure for the hospital assistant within the service, we have created promotional posts for them. These posts are based on workload, responsibility, the geography of the country, and so on. For example, at the district hospital level, the post of senior hospital assistant was created. At the larger general hospital level, there is a third grade, the chief hospital assistant.

The newly graduated hospital assistants are first posted for one or two years at larger establishments where their work can be supervised. They are then transferred to remote areas for two years. At the end of this period, they have gained sufficient experience to go to a larger town or to be deployed to public health programmes to work in malaria, tuberculosis or leprosy control. After six or seven years, they may be promoted to the senior grade at district hospitals. From there, selected individuals may go on to become chief hospital assistant. This career structure provides increased remuneration and also provides opportunities for the children of these officers to go from primary to secondary and then to high school without having been separated from their parents. We find this is very important if we want to keep hospital assistants in the service.

So far we have been successful in making use of hospital assistants. The reason is because a specific place has been found for them in the government health service that provides them with the necessary security enjoyed by civil servants. They are not allowed to set up independent practice outside the government services.

DU GAS (*Canada*): I have mentioned that we are developing nurse practitioners rather than physician's assistants. This solves a a lot of problems, but we believe

that in developing career patterns for these nurses, it is extremely important to maintain flexibility so that nurses may proceed from one level to another. We think that the nurse practitioner should be allowed to come to this field from either a registered nurse diploma programme or a baccalaureate nursing programme and that the preparatory programme should carry university credit.

To attract and retain people, not only nurses but also physicians and other health workers, in the rural and remote areas of Canada's North, we are setting up a scholarship programme. People who work in the North for two years can receive a one-year university scholarship with full pay.

One province provides a guaranteed income for physicians in underserved areas. If the physician's earnings do not reach this level, the government supplements them.

ACUÑA (*Mexico*): The problem of the status of personnel affects all—the physician, the nurse, and the auxiliary personnel. In Mexico, for example, until very recently, the ideal of a student of medicine was to become a specialist as soon as possible. This trend is changing somewhat, and we are hearing more about the general practitioner, a family doctor with certain postgraduate training. The same urge for specialization also affects the field of nursing. The nurse is not satisfied with a degree in nursing. She wants a higher professional status and income and, therefore, aspires to become a nurse paediatrician, surgical nurse, or other specialist. This same tendency is also seen at the lower levels of health assistant and sanitary officer.

Medical assistants are selected by the local community health committee, and naturally they have ambitions. We hope that as part of the system of rewards for this type of personnel, it may prove possible to offer fellowships for completion of secondary schooling and, later, nursing studies. It is important to emphasize here that the majority of rural populations have a dual culture— the indigenous native influence and the western culture derived from colonial times. Thus, the person selected for training as a medical assistant should feel at home in his dual culture and thus be able both to interpret the community needs and to understand modern medicine.

Undoubtedly the status of the assistant, once he is trained and working, will be high in the community by virtue of his recognition by the state health authorities. On the other hand, this improved status at community level would, of course, be lost if the individual desired to look further afield in the larger area of the regional health services, where he would obviously start at the lowest rung.

TABIBZADEH (*Iran*): I believe that a long-range career status for this type of personnel and the ability to retain their services for a long period of time are goals that can be achieved only if they work within the structure of a health delivery system.

For example, in a health network the small rural health centre must be connected to health centres, and each health centre must be connected to the larger specialized health centres. These specialized health centres must, in turn, be connected to the general hospital, which relates to certain completely specialized institutions.

If there is no unified and interconnected system of health delivery, then each individual unit really functions in a vacuum and the career status of these people will be gradually lost. But if they are inside a system they can, after a few years at one level and with a little additional training, move to higher positions.

MINKOLA-NDOSIMAU (*Zaire*): In my earlier remarks on the training and recruitment of medical assistants in my country, I mentioned the suspension of programmes. There are two aspects to this; one professional and the other administrative.

Professionally, the medical assistants are intermediate level personnel who remain in that category. They are neither doctors nor nurses and cannot aspire to promotion or engage in activities reserved for the doctor.

Administratively, all careers within the public administration are under the Ministry of Public Administration. Our functions fall under this department and not under that of National Education. But certain requirements must be met for positions within the public service and these requirements are established by the Ministry of National Education. Our paramedical personnel—nurses and medical auxiliaries—found themselves caught between these administrative and educational requirements. Individuals in administrative careers could progress up the administrative ladder, but this was not true for paramedical personnel, who were left without a channel for advancement.

At the present time, the concern of health authorities centres on finding a formula that will allow the paramedical and nursing categories an opportunity of honourable progress and promotion within the profession. This is made somewhat difficult by the centralization of administration. Under the 1971 reform of the university system, all areas pertaining to higher education became the responsibility of the national university. Previously, the country had three universities. These have now become campuses of one central university. There is now only one school of medicine and it is responsible for education in all paramedical fields. It is also responsible for studying these problems together with the Ministry of Public Health.

BATHKE (*USA*): It has been my experience that the 'system' must include career development. One method would be the development of a career lattice that comprehends all health careers.

In rural or developing areas, because of the shortage of educated and qualified personnel, administrative programmes often tend to recruit from other sectors, such as health careers. Consequently, upon completion of their training, physicians or physician's assistants are often recruited into administrative programmes. While this is not necessarily a waste of their education, it does not use it to the fullest, because the people in the community are still without a doctor of a physician's assistant.

Therefore, to preserve the career status of the physician's assistant, we must also encourage the development of separate and distinct health administration careers.

WATSON (*Papua New Guinea*): An administrative career is, unfortunately, often the most lucrative one. If you close that door to people, you will not be their friend. I believe that promotion should come most readily to those who stay in the role for which they have been trained and who perform well. If there is a grade 1, grade 2, grade 3 system, there should be more grade 2 positions relative to grade 1 (base grade) positions in the field for which a person has been trained. There should not be a high proportion of grade 2 positions in specialized sections such as tuberculosis, leprosy, malaria, administration, health education, and so on. We have not achieved that in Papua New Guinea; in fact, we have the opposite situation! I see this as a real need.

We have no promotional scale for our lower grade doctor auxiliary, the aid post orderly. Many of these workers, partly because they have no career, are quite demoralized.

I share Fendall's view that there should be a career structure within any category to give the person job satisfaction and a goal to work towards. He should not, of course, be constantly wishing to move from his category into a different one, for example, that of the medical officer.

However, it should be possible—possible but very difficult—for a medical assistant to pass from one category to the other. In Papua New Guinea, it should be theoretically possible for our lowest person, the aid post orderly, to pass up through the ranks of medical assistant (health extension officer) and on to become a doctor. He could do this only by raising his own level of basic education and by showing real promise. This has never happened, but I believe we would have a healthier service if there were a few individuals who had done this.

FLAHAULT (*WHO, Geneva*): It think that it is not a pure coincidence that the first speaker on the question of careers was from Iran, which is a country that has had certain difficulties in the training of the medical assistants precisely because the problem of careers had not been carefully considered beforehand. This led, in many cases, to the failure of programmes. I believe that we should consider this question in connection with that of the careers of the other members of the health team. Today the Soviet Union is probably the country that uses medical assistants in the best possible way. Sidel, who modestly has referred to the work he has carried out in the area of the feldsher in the USSR, could tell us about their position in the Soviet Union.

SIDEL (*USA*): With specific regard to career mobility, relatively few feldshers climb the career ladder to become physicians. If the feldsher is in the top 5 % of his graduating class, there is indeed the possibility of his moving into medical school immediately or very soon after graduation. He begins back at the start of medical education, so far as I can tell, and requires the full six years, but he has a somewhat easier time with his studies. If he does not do this very shortly after his graduation, the chances for it diminish, and apparently it happens quite rarely.

With respect to status, the feldsher who originally came from the rural village in which he practises has a fair degree of status in the village. This not rarely happens. There are few doctors, and the feldsher achieves status by becoming educated and returning in an important health role.

On the other hand, if the feldsher does not come from the village where he practises, or if he is working in an area in which there are physicians, it is reported that status problems do indeed arise. It is no accident that the word 'feldsherism' in the Soviet Union has come to mean something that is second rate or an inadequate copy of another kind of role. But the Soviet literature separates the feldsher, who is judged to do an excellent job, from the concept of 'feldsherism'.

There are great differences, of course, between the role of the feldsher in the rural areas, where he often works relatively independently, and his role in the cities, where he works closely with other health workers. The role of the feldsher in the USSR changes as needs change and as more and more physicians are trained, but it remains an important one.

SMITH (*USA*): I would like to give some perspective to Dr Sidel's remarks as they relate to the developing world. And in this case, as far as health care is concerned, that must include the United States.

We must look at how long the system of feldshers has been in operation in the Soviet Union, the purpose for which it was developed, and what accounts for the downgrading of feldsherism in the USSR. This may partly reflect the recent emphasis on the production of large numbers of physicians. In the rest of the world, we must ask ourselves whether we have an adequate number of physicians where needed before we examine in a very narrow way the history of the Soviet feldsher. The feldshers performed a huge and necessary task for the Soviet Union during a very trying development period.

In our period, we must find some answers which, though not feldsherism, may be something equally different for our own communities. At the same time, we must understand some of the reasons for the beginning of the possible disappearance of the felsher in Russia.

SIDEL (*USA*): The latest figures suggest that the doctor–patient ratio in the Soviet Union is approaching one physician for every 400 people. The USSR has a very much larger ratio of physicians, and, therefore, a very different role for its physicians than is found in the countries represented around the table, including the United States. It is no surprise that the feldsher's role is also different. What is surprising and exciting is that USSR has taken an old role, developed in response to scarce manpower, and modified and strengthened it in response to new needs.

HAKIM (*Sudan*): I think the stability of career status depends entirely on the appreciation of that status. We consider the medical assistant to be the backbone of our health services. This gives trainees the psychological and the practical support and stability which has sustained this cadre of health workers for the last 50 years. Adding to the stability of the cadre is their acceptance by the population for whom they work and the mutual confidence that exists between them and the sectors of population remote from a physician's attention.

In our early experience, some medical assistants tried to profit from the confidence of their people and attempted to carry out private practice as doctors. This endangered the stability of career status and we had to combat it during the training period by giving trainees instruction on the definition of their role, and on their functions and duties.

The stability of these workers has also been strengthened by giving them satisfactory remuneration. Further, we offer them postgraduate courses. Some of them are trained to become anaesthetists or pharmacists. Refresher courses are an effective way of stimulating their interest. We also give the most senior medical assistants special training so that they can do some training themselves. Some senior posts are administrative and this is appropriate. Some take posts in which they inspect the work of others and help them to gain a better understanding of patients and how to manage them. The physicians themselves have helped to stabilize the career of this cadre by making tours to areas for which they are responsible.

ESTES (*USA*): Dr Flahault has emphasized the necessity for a team role. I want to pursue that point briefly.

In any team there must be a leader, and there must be followers. We have had several students in our physician's assistant programme who could have entered medical school if they had so chosen. They actually preferred to have a secondary role in the team as a follower rather than as a leader. As a matter of fact, we have one student who has already completed the required work for the medical degree. Despite our efforts to persuade him to become a doctor, he is quite serious in his preference to remain a physician's assistant.

In dealing with medical students and doctors, we have sometimes forgotten that there are those who do not want primary responsibility or to be the team leader.

FERNANDO (*Ceylon*): I think we should differentiate between status and career. Status refers to a state or circumstance attached to a particular job rather than the specific characteristics of the job. I think the background factors for status are the entrance requirements for securing a post and the quality of the training undergone. The higher the entrance requirements and the longer the period of training, the greater would be the status. Status will be different depending upon whether the curriculum is general or specialized. The skills acquired and the responsibilities undertaken will be different.

If we arrange our training programmes in the best way and in stages, would it not be possible for the medical assistant, trained for one year, to receive a few more years of training so that he can keep moving up the ladder? To the question whether he can become a doctor, we say no. But we should work out a scheme or lattice, whereby he can move in his own branch, as well as move into other branches, within that lattice.

Someone mentioned that the MEDEX should be satisfied with their career status. Dissatisfaction always comes later. After serving in a certain position for some time, there may be no place to go. That is the point at which you should ask people whether they are satisfied.

CONANT (*USA*): In nursing we have had experience in this area that might be helpful. Over the years the best nurses have tended to move out of nursing practice into administrative and teaching positions. The result has been that the quality of nursing care has not improved.

It is important to have built-in incentives to encourage people to improve their practice while remaining practitioners. If the only way that people can receive recognition and better salaries is by becoming administrators, the most able will tend to leave practice for administration.

TADELLE (*Ethiopia*): I would like to add something to what Professor Fernando said regarding the educational opportunities for medical assistants. Educational opportunities should be open to able and qualified medical assistants. Usually, the argument against this has reflected the particular interest of professional or other groups; the correct perspective has been disregarded.

Regular salary increments and financial incentives are very difficult to provide in many countries. In order to promote job satisfaction, it is therefore even more necessary to give educational opportunities to able medical assistants.

Among other factors, the attrition rate of the medical assistant has got to be considered in any career scheme. One of the arguments is that, if given advanced training, medical assistants would leave the work they are trained for, and could no longer be retained in rural areas. But it is logical and natural for anyone without a defined career to aspire to better working conditions.

In summary then, concerning career schemes and other educational opportunities, the medical assistant has to be considered on equal grounds with other health professionals.

DIESH (*India*): In order to avoid stagnation and frustration, we have opened promotional avenues in the hierarchy of the health structure of our country. We place the junior community worker with nine months training, what we call the basic health worker, in the rural areas to cover a population of 10 000; he is helped by an auxillary nurse midwife who is his female counterpart.

Above this, there is a health assistant and a health visitor (female) for 40 000 population, covering four of the peripheral units. At the next higher level, the primary health centre level, the senior health assistant and public health nurse work for a population of 80 000–100 000.

This is an attempt to provide sufficient promotional channels for people employed at the different administrative levels.

Another attempt to provide promotional avenues has been made by introducing the degree of Bachelor of Science in Public Health (B.Sc.P.H.). With this qualification, it is possible to rise to the district level as senior health supervisor, or to be placed as junior health officer at the subdivisional level where there are no health officers at present.

We are now convinced that health assistants should be recruited from the locality to which they will return to work. I entirely agree with the delegate from Iran that introduction of the MEDEX system should be very carefully considered. Our experience is that 'half-baked doctors' are a danger to health. I am sure that if we introduce the MEDEX system, every MEDEX will desire to become a doctor.

MINKOLA-NDOSIMAU (*Zaire*): I wish to ask whether our colleagues from the USA could give us some idea of the promotional opportunities for the category of medical assistant. I would like also to know how the medical assistant here is integrated into the health team. I did not fully understand what are his relationships with other members of the medical team, particularly the nurse.

ESTES (*USA*): Regarding avenues for promotion within the health structure in the USA, we have not had any graduate assistants from our programme enter medical school, but we have had an American Indian student who dropped out of our programme after one year to enter medical school.

I agree that there should always be an opportunity for the ambitious individual to move ahead. The medical school route is very difficult because it is highly competitive, and I think very few will be successful in gaining admission.

There is another available avenue. Two of our graduates have entered a school of public health and obtained master's degrees in public health. Both have entered the health care planning area. Other graudates have entered medical educational careers through joining other training programmes.

The relationship between assistants and nurses depends on the setting. We utilize both physician's assistants and nurse practitioners in a clinical setting where they work side by side doing precisely the same work. There is no distinction.

SILVER (*USA*): As I mentioned earlier, the child health associate receives a bachelor's degree on completion of the first two years in the programme and is eligible for a master's degree on completion of the third year. In our school, as in other schools, it is now possible to apply some of the basic science courses that are taken prior to entering the child health associate programme.

None of our graduates has wanted to go to medical school, but they could move in that direction if they desired.

In some settings, nurse practitioners and child health associates work very well together. The child health associate can diagnose and treat, and may write prescriptions for a large variety of drugs. His is a much more extensive role than that of the nurse practitioner. The nurse practitioner may work in a doctor's office, in a public health facility under a doctor's supervision, or in a health station or other public health facility some distance from a physician who may visit only once a week or even less.

SMITH (*USA*): By inventing a new name, simply by beginning to create an identity for a totally new profession, we were able to do things we thought might not have been possible. We intend to build a profession that provides a professionally satisfying career. As Dr Estes and Dr Silver have indicated, none of us has had problems in integrating MEDEX into the present health care system with nurses or physicians.

Approximately 20% of the MEDEX trainees thought at entry that they wanted to go to medical school. Thus far, of nearly 300 who have graduated, only one has gone on to medical school; he did so at the insistence of the physicians with whom he worked. Most of the MEDEX feel very confident that they have found a satisfying career. Their average is about 29, and at that stage they do not want to spend time in going on to medical school. The youngest we have ever taken was 22; he was the one who went to medical school.

Seventy-five percent of the MEDEX have remained in rural areas. As far as mobility is concerned, at least 25% have moved out of their original training site, with no difficulty.

To summarize the discussion, I believe that integration of the medical assistant into a system in the public sector becomes paramount, particularly as it relates to rural areas. The system must have built-in mechanisms for growth, such as continuing education and a progression of salaries and opportunities. These are probably the most critical elements for strengthening the career of the medical assistant.

Our participant from Togo spoke about how their training programme provides satisfying careers for people who are dissatisfied with their jobs. In many instances we encounter such people who are simply under-utilized, especially by those of us who are physicians. Physicians have not yet learned how to utilize all the people in the health care team. Specialized cadres may also provide additional satisfying roles within a career category.

As Dr Hardin mentioned, continuation in this career in areas of need may depend upon factors which also affect the staying power of physicians and nurses in rural areas or in city centres. Perhaps some of these same factors should be considered in the training of medical assistants, but I would prefer that such planning be done before rather than after the individual has been trained.

Mr Bathke's description of medical assistants moving into administrative roles should not be taken lightly because there are many instances of very competent people who are needed as providers of health care being lost in that way.

I would call your attention to page 13 of Dr Flahault's article[1] in *World Health* which gives an outline of a medical assistant's career somewhat similar to those that we heard about this afternoon. It serves as an apparently very workable model and one which fits the thinking of most of us who have been actively involved in training medical assistants.

Dr Watson said that mobility upward should be made difficult but not impossible. This has implications which should be considered and understood.

Mobility and planning for career status should be an integral part of the short-range as well as the long-range planning for any career development strategy for the medical assistant.

The critical issue that we face in common, however, is to find successful methods for providing health services to populations which have no access or limited access to care. The development of career status, as we have stated time and time again, requires special attention at all stages of planning these programmes.

---

[1] Flahault, D. (1972) The case for medical assistants. *World Health*, June, pp. 8–15.

120

ACCEPTANCE, PUBLIC AND PROFESSIONAL

Chairman: VICTOR W. SIDEL, M.D.[1]

Moderator: MALCOLM TODD, M.D.[2]

TODD (*USA*): I have been impressed by the presentations of the representatives of the many countries participating in this Conference. I am sure that none can leave with the impression that we in the USA have solved the problems under discussion. Quite the opposite is true! It was only eight or nine years ago that the physician's assistant concept was started at Duke University, followed by the MEDEX programmes, and Dr Silver's programmes. Our experience is indeed short and, in many respects, not necessarily applicable to other nations.

I suggest that we discuss acceptance or non-acceptance by the public and by the profession as manifested in some objective surveys and in the personal experience that each of you has had with developing programmes. It might be more useful to examine acceptance by first considering the factors that contribute to non-acceptance.

There is a real lack of understanding on the part of many individuals about the entire concept of the medical assistant. The wide variety of programmes—physician associate, MEDEX, primex, nurse practitioner, paediatric nurse associate, paediatric nurse assistant, etc.—has tended to confuse the public about the purposes and place of medical assistants. A facet that has not been touched upon here is non-acceptance by the individuals who reside in the inner cities, in the ghetto areas of some of our metropolitan communities. In the recent development of comprehensive health planning in the USA, a number of conferences have been held with citizens and community groups who are interested in the provision of health care. These people are very vocal; they are very vehement in rejecting what they regard as second-rate, substandard care.

Dr Alfred Haynes, who is director of the MEDEX programme at the Drew Medical School in Los Angeles, has found this to be one of his major problems. But he is finding answers and will overcome this obstacle. Dr Sidel has mentioned the concern about substandard care in the feldsher system. These examples indicate that we must be careful to avoid creating either the impression or the fact of two standards of care.

Another factor in non-acceptance has been the rivalry between nurses and physician's assistants—and the rivalries between midwives and obstetricians, between the obstetrician nurse practitioners and the obstetricians and between the various nurse midwifery programmes themselves.

---

[1] Montefiore Hospital, Bronx, New York.
[2] American Medical Association, Council on Health Manpower, Long Beach, California.

There are also problems concerning the employment of medical assistants. In the USA, institutions are probably going to be the primary source of employment for these trained individuals.

There are, therefore, many facets to the whole concept of the medical assistant that must be carefully considered at the outset so that difficulties may be anticipated and circumvented by planning.

One of our major concerns has been the lack of the primary care physician. By primary care physician, I mean a family practitioner, an internist, a paediatrician, and even an obstetrician. These are individuals who have the principal control of the patient's care as he moves through the system.

Much of our medical education has been geared to specialization without adequate regard to supply and demand. There are, for example, too many general surgeons in the USA. That brings us to the category of the subspecialty physician's assistant, the orthopaedic assistant, and the urologist assistant. There are surgeons in some universities who feel that there is a need for a surgical physician's assistant.

The Duke University programme, which was designed to fill the gap in medical care in medically deprived and rural areas, is a laudable one. A great deal of progress has been made. But the fact is that some of its graduates have chosen to stay in the cities with a busy practitioner who can then have more time off from his practice. In addition, some of these excellently trained assistants have chosen to teach in physician's assistant programmes, or have gone into other states to set up or assist physicians's assistant activities and programmes. Thus, there is a difference of opinion about how effectively this new source of manpower is meeting the need and how best they can be utilized in the future.

I conclude by emphasizing our basic concern to develop the role of the primary care physician in our own system.

GORIUP (*Algeria*): In Africa during the colonial period, work in the field of health was concentrated on mass campaigns against communicable diseases, and numerous medical assistants were trained mainly for that purpose.

Independence coincided more or less with the attainment of the consolidation phase in the control of many diseases, with more emphasis laid on personal care, such as that provided by medical practitioners. The attitude of the government became less favourable to the medical auxiliaries and their training was slowed down or stopped.

When it became generally accepted that epidemiological surveillance and personal care had to be extended to the rural areas and the concept of basic health services gained more and more favour, the need for medical auxiliaries was again felt. Yet the medical and nursing professions do not readily accept this new type of health worker, sometimes considered as a potential competitor.

This difficulty could be overcome if the functions of the medical auxiliaries within the health team were better defined and were well known to the rest of its members.

In Algeria, an effort to achieve this goal is made by training medical students, student nurses and medical assistants together in rural health centres. It is hoped that better understanding and improved relations within health teams will result in the future.

VILLARREAL (*PAHO, Washington, D.C.*): I wish to refer briefly to two studies in Latin America related to the delegation of functions to auxiliary personnel.

One of these studies was carried out in Colombia in close collaboration with the Government of that country, the Association of Colombian Schools of

Medicine, and the Pan American Health Organization. The study carefully analysed community acceptance of the services provided by this type of auxiliary personnel. It showed the results to have been extremely satisfactory and to have demonstrated the unreserved acceptance of auxiliary personnel by the people benefiting from their services. Some of the activities performed by auxiliaries were compared with those carried out by physicians. There were no significant differences in the way in which these activities were carried out.

In Cuba, a broad programme has been undertaken to train auxiliary personnel including dental care personnel (stomatologists and dental assistants). This type of personnel has been widely accepted by the community, and some 500 auxiliaries have been trained and are providing dental care in Cuba.

BEAUSOLEIL (*Ghana*): I disagree with some points raised by Dr Goriup. In Ghana, for example, auxiliary health workers have been used for well over 50 years and are accepted by the Government, professionals, and the public. It is understood that auxiliaries will continue to render valuable services for a long time to come; our concern now is to improve their quality.

A problem arises, however, in those areas where the felt needs of the community cannot be met by the auxiliary health worker and there is a consequent demand for the services of the professional. This demand is not easy to meet, and considerable efforts are made to resist it because of the need to utilize the auxiliary in providing basic health services and to keep the services of the professional for those tasks that cannot be delegated. This is necessary because of an acute shortage of trained personnel, particularly at the professional level.

However, in those special areas where the demand for the services of the professional is justified, efforts are being made to provide them. This has become possible because of the availability of relatively large numbers of young physicians who cannot be placed in hospitals because of lack of accommodation. These physicians are to be given suitable orientation to prepare them for rural health work.

Our experience is that, even where there is a professional, the auxiliary is still accepted, although invariably the professional is more acceptable than the auxiliary.

TABIBZADEH (*Iran*): We must study the felt needs of the population in order to increase acceptance. For example, when in the early period of the malaria programme we did spraying operations, probably the poorly educated rural population did not understand what caused malaria, but when they saw that the mosquitos and flies had been reduced, their acceptance increased. While we were in a consolidation phase and taking blood smears, there was no acceptance because the people did not understand the reason for it and did not feel the need for it.

In a developing country where the public health problems are great and emphasis is on prevention, the rate of acceptance is usually very low. We must train medical assistants in a mixture of preventive and curative medicine in order to meet the felt need of the population in remote areas.

EL HAKIM (*Sudan*): In considering acceptance, we have to consider four aspects. First is the national or official acceptance. Since we consider the medical assistant as the backbone of our rural services, he is officially accepted.

The second aspect concerns the physician. The physician plays a very important role in the selection and training of the medical assistant. He also works with him, either as his supervisor, or on the cases referred from him, or in giving him postgraduate or refresher courses. Hence, if the physician is carrying out all these duties connected with the medical assistant, he invariably finds the assistant acceptable.

The third aspect of acceptance relates to other auxiliary disciplines. The medical assistant works with a health visitor in dispensaries, and with a midwife and other auxiliaries in the health centre. Hence, they work as a small team in places where a physician's services may not be available. The medical assistant is accepted by these classes of auxiliaries.

The fourth aspect concerns acceptance by the public. This is rather delicate because other factors are involved. The medical assistant generally comes from the population of the area and hence is known to the people. In most cases, they seem to like him as a person. But the public will demand more services as time goes on. They may not entirely rely on the medical assistant as the years pass. In ten years their reliance may be placed rather on a medical officer or physician. In the future, care must be taken to teach medical assistants at a fairly high level to cope with the demands and requests of the public.

Acceptance by all segments of society is generally a good measure of the success of a programme; lack of acceptance indicates the opposite and may cause the whole system to collapse.

In our country, for the time being, acceptance is general, indicating that the system is strong and should continue for the next few years. As educators we should ensure that the standards of our medical assistants gradually improve as time goes on to meet new needs and demands. Continued general acceptance will reflect the strength and effectiveness of this group of medical workers.

NATHANIELS (*Togo*): The acceptance of medical assistants must be considered from several different points of view. It depends in a great measure on the medical assistant himself, i.e., his competence. He must behave like a qualified and capable professional man. He should neither have a superiority complex vis-à-vis the lower level auxiliary personnel nor an inferiority complex towards the higher staff. He must be conscious of the fact that he has to integrate himself fully into the system of health care. It is during the course of his training that he should acquire these attitudes.

Second, the school that prepares the medical assistant must share the responsibility for his acceptance or otherwise. The school should prepare him to succeed, and we, as teachers, must provide the right kind of education. I suggest that we should include individual and social psychology in our programme.

Third is public acceptance. Here again, the medical assistant should assume responsibility for his competence both in health work and in his relations with the public. In the rural areas, as Dr Flahault pointed out earlier, he would be the well-informed counsellor, hence the inclusion in our programme of the rudiments of law.

Fourth is physician acceptance. Medical doctors are not yet persuaded of the utility of the medical assistant, but I believe this situation will improve. Efforts are required from both the school and the student to promote acceptance. The former must provide a suitable education, and the latter should aim for proficiency from the outset of his training.

I emphasize again the need for a good system of education, appropriate to the circumstances. I believe Duke University is in the vanguard of such educational efforts. We are not going to copy their programme exactly but will adapt teaching methods to the conditions prevailing in our country. Emphasis will be placed on preventive medicine.

JACKSON (*USA*): The medical assistant has been around for a long time. We called her our Girl Friday or our handyman. Patients liked the medical assistant. If they did not like the medical assistant, they did not come back to the doctor.

One of the things I did not hear discussed in the last two days is the matter of medical records. If more attention were given to having medical assistants help the doctors in keeping the medical records, especially with the current development of aids such as tape recorders, this would free the doctor to provide more services to the patients.

SOOPIKIAN (*Iran*): I will confine myself to acceptance in the public sector, because in our part of the world we use this type of auxiliary mostly in the public sector. We have a more or less standardized type of health system with graded health centres connected to district and regional hospitals.

In rural health centres we previously used the medical assistant but we do so no longer. Now lower level auxiliaries work with doctors in such centres. Our studies show that one must provide an even distribution of doctors in rural areas. If not, people in an area without a doctor are not happy about taking a lower grade auxiliary instead, although they will accept such a person rather than have nothing. We are planning to introduce a new and lower level of auxiliary rather than a medical assistant for small and remote populations. The MEDEX approach is not suitable for us if the MEDEX does no more than assist the physician in his private clinical practice. In our part of the world help for the urban doctor is not the main problem.

When we speak of acceptance, this means acceptance of the total system by the population. Even this system with strategic placement of doctors and specialists is frequently bypassed by people unless they must follow it to obtain insurance payments. People will bypass rural doctors, who represent 22% of Iran's doctors, and go to a more qualified physician or specialist, or else to hospital outpatient departments. They do this even when care in the public sector is given free or for a nominal charge.

In the Soviet Union, there are district doctors who are the first point of referral. People cannot see another doctor unless they first go through the district doctor. That is not the case in our country.

So we have difficulty with the whole system. We planners provide for coverage of different groups of people in what appears to be a very comprehensive and satisfactory system, but the people will not follow that system.

We have both a public and a private medical system in Iran. It is interesting to note that people quite often shift from public to private institutions, particularly for ambulatory care. So acceptance really must reflect acceptance of the total system by the population.

TADELLE (*Ethiopia*): Acceptance of medical assistants, expecially in the rural areas of the developing world, has to be seen in relation to the traditional practitioners who are part of the existing reality. The performance of the medical assistant is a vital factor in his acceptance in such context.

Acceptance may not be a problem in areas where modern medicine has never been introduced. In such places, any type of health worker will be accepted until the people come to realize the existence and availability of better qualified practitioners. Hence, acceptance should be considered in relation to the literacy of the people, geographical location, etc.

There is also acceptance through identification of the type of health worker with the institution in which he is expected to work. For instance, a medical assistant is expected to work in a clinic, a doctor is supposed to practise within a hospital setting, and so on.

With regard to professional acceptance, I would only say that the ability of medical assistants to perform diagnoses is underestimated by physicians. Therefore, the attitude of physicians may influence acceptance either positively or negatively.

MINKOLA-NDOSIMAU (*Zaire*): In our country the category of medical assistant has been known for a long time. Since 1936 we have had schools to train these people. The acceptance of medical care given by the medical assistant varies with the individual, and it varies in the rural and urban environments.

In the past, the medical assistants have proved themselves in practice, and they have been accepted. But there are some hesitations in the urban areas. For example, some problems arise with people of high rank who prefer to see a physician, whereas people at a lower socioeconomic level may see a medical assistant who, they know, is not a full-fledged doctor. In the rural areas, the medical assistant is at the summit of the medical profession and people will certainly go to him.

The acceptance of the medical assistant by the population depends on the environment—rural or urban—and the circumstances under which he is working. The length of time that modern medicine has been introduced in a country is also a factor in acceptance.

ACUÑA (*Mexico*): Some doubt has been expressed in regard to the acceptance of health services by the population. I believe that the people would not only accept them but demand them. As far as Mexico is concerned, there is certainly a demand on the part of the rural population for improved health services, particularly medical services. Various systems have been tried and different methods have been taught. We believe that certain systems and services have been rejected when they have been managed by outside persons who do not have a great interest in a job which they know they are doing for only a short period. Thus there must be emphasis on the use of local people who are known to and identified with the community.

Acceptance has also been studied in other spheres in Mexico. At the moment, health care services are provided by the Mexican Social Security Institute, which covers about 30% of the population, mainly in urban areas. The Government and state health services take care of the rest, except for the relatively small part of the population able to afford the services of private practitioners and hospitals. A certain amount of resistance to the institutionalized and public services has been evident.

Our medical schools have stressed specialization to such an extent that these services have a large percentage of specialized medical personnel but lack general practitioners and family doctors. So, in many instances, the first contact the patient has with medical personnel is not with the general practitioner but with the specialist. The specialist finds that the disease from which the patient suffers does not fall within his specialty, and so the patient is referred to another doctor. The patient opposes the idea of seeing a specialist before going through the filter of the general practitioner or family doctor.

DIESH (*India*): Each country has to have a pattern and structure of health care related to its own health needs. There cannot be one single international standard. What is true in New York City or in New Delhi may not be valid in Madras or Las Vegas. In developing countries like ours, an attempt should be made to produce doctors with a basic training and well equipped to serve in the rural areas.

The physician–patient relationship is a very personal one and has a major role to play in providing health services to the community. We have seen what may happen in a hospital. There may be three doctors, of whom two are sitting idle while patients wait in a long queue to see the third. A great deal depends upon the doctor's ability and behaviour and his feeling for the patient. But in areas where there are no doctors, even a paramedical or a quack is accepted because he renders some kind of medical aid.

We are not inclined to follow what is done in some countries and use the paramedical workers as full-fledged doctors. Wherever they are employed, they should work under the guidance and supervision of a qualified doctor.

WATSON (*Papua New Guinea*): I would like to support those who have said that people who have nothing will accept anything. I wish to be more positive, however.

The second year of health extension officer training includes a little sociology. Trainees spend from two weeks to a month living in a village with an aid post. They are required to find out, both by observation and by asking, what the people think of the aid post, of the subdistrict hospital and of the district hospital. The district hospital, in this particular case, is a $2 million disaster. I view it as a disaster because it uses something like three-quarters of that district's total allocation of funds.

The people generally are very grateful for the aid post. They are less sure about the subdistrict hospital, and they are quite antagonistic toward the district hospital. We see this in practice, too. People who need transfer to the subdistrict hospital from the aid post are reluctant. And people in the subdistrict hospital who need transfer to the district hospital often refuse to go.

We also see people who bypass the aid post. Even the least sophisticated of people are able to be selective. They like to have a service close by for the things they regard as relatively unimportant, but if they believe something needs 'more important treatment,' they will go and get that 'more important treatment.'

SIDEL (*USA*): I would like to comment on what Dr Todd said about my being concerned that the feldshers in the USSR delivered 'substandard care.' This is not correct. What I said in my writings on the feldsher is that some people in the Soviet Union have commented that individual feldshers have at times not delivered optimal care for certain specific conditions. In general, the health services leadership in the Soviet Union, the physicians, the feldshers themselves, and their patients seem quite happy with the role being played by the feldshers.

On the other hand, there are reports that the Soviet Union is increasingly trying to phase out the independent role of the feldsher and to train more doctors relative to the number of feldshers being trained. What is unclear to me is to what extent this policy is based upon a critical evaluation of the role of the feldsher and to what extent it is based on what one might call 'national pride', an aversion to the use of what observers in other countries might consider to be 'second-class' medical personnel.

When we talk about acceptance, therefore, I think we have to talk not only about acceptance and professional acceptance, but also about acceptance by society and national pride. The resistance to the medical assistant may be 'irrational' in the sense that it is a resistance to an ill-understood name, ideology, or concept, rather than resistance to a specific job description or to a specific well-trained well-supervised worker who provides certain services not only as well as in some ways even better than does the physician.

TODD (*USA*): I think we will all agree that the comments made by Dr Watson, Dr Diesh, and Dr Soopikian are extremely significant as reflecting ideas and attitudes encountered in their countries.

We must concede that the acceptance of this level of health worker varies in different settings and situations. There is not one uniform pattern that will accommodate all variations. Certainly, there is a difference between acceptance in the private sector and acceptance in the public sector. While the USA has not yet moved to a nationalized health system, there are many who believe this is not far away. Probably costs will be the most important deterrent to such a programme.

The acceptance of this level of health worker by the professional and by other health workers also varies. It is true that in some communities the public has accepted them almost with open arms.

I would like to comment again on Dr Smith's MEDEX programme in the State of Washington. There is the example of the two young MEDEX who go 40 miles from Spokane to a community of 1800 people which had never had a doctor, and work under the guidance of a physician in Spokane. These two men take an active part in the affairs to that community, they are liked by the people and the community will want to keep them. This is acceptance. But we must be concerned about what happens if the doctor preceptor dies. We will need to have preceptors to substitute for that individual under the system that has been presented.

I should comment on the health team that many of you have mentioned. The health team may be of two types. Probably the basic type is the team consisting of the doctor and his nurse, a technician, and now perhaps a physician's assistant. This unit can be expanded to a health team that would also include a dentist, hospital administrators, social workers, technicians of various types, and community health workers. There will be a place, of course, for this type of health team in providing health care in the USA, and I am sure we will go through the same experiences as many of you have had in your own countries.

I do not think it makes much difference who is captain of the team. There are many doctors who have ability in administration and in providing leadership. A doctor who has this ability should be captain of the team. On the other hand, there are doctors who know nothing about administration. In some circumstances, therefore, a hospital administrator would make a better administrative officer of the health team. We have to be open-minded about who is going to be captain of the health team. In all cases, it must be an individual who has the force and capacity to give directions, and make the health team function as it should.

From the discussion, you might think that we have 10 000 to 12 000 of these workers in the field in the USA today. That is not true. As of December 1972, we had 51 approved programmes. Questionnaires were sent to all the programme directors and 50 responded. Twenty of the schools or programme had no graduates at all. There was a total of 585 graduates of whom 461 were working as assistants to physicians. Of those, 236 were working in doctor's offices and 225 were working in institutional settings.

In June 1973 this figure will move up rapidly, and there will probably be approximately 800 to 900 graduates of the various schools by the end of the year.

ASSURANCE OF QUALITY, COMPETENCE, AND ACCOUNTABILITY

ACCREDITATION

by WILLIAM K. SELDEN, Ph.D.[1]

At this session I have been asked to speak on what is frequently considered a rather prosaic subject—accreditation. I plan to pass in review some of the social factors that have been involved in this peculiar development of control of educational programmes in the USA. Peculiar, I say, because it is found nowhere else, although attempts have been made to introduce certain features of this system in the Philippines, and an abortive attempt was made after the Second World War to establish a form of accreditation in Japan.

To understand accreditation, which I will shortly define, we must recall that in the early years of the development of the USA we did rely considerably on apprentice training for people in the medical and health professions, and that our early schools and colleges were largely sponsored by religious denominations, primarily, but not exclusively, protestant.

When the Constitution of the United States of America was developed in the late eighteenth century, these factors were taken into account, and education was considered to be a state responsibility. As a result, responsibility for education was dispersed among the initial 13 states.

There is considerable variation among the states in their attitudes regarding responsibility and legislation for education. Consequently, education has not been developed as a national operation or with major national policies. Furthermore, in the nineteenth century, we actually rescinded certain state laws dealing with licensure. And during the second third of the past century, partially in response to the frontier influence of the country, a very marked laissez-faire attitude prevailed in economic and social matters.

If was in these circumstances that recognition was given to the need to establish some kind of regulation over standards of education. Accreditation was developed by the educational institutions themselves to meet a need of society that the Government was not prepared to provide.

Within the same historical context the professions, led by medicine, assumed prerogatives with respect to the educational development of their

---

[1] National Commission on Accrediting, Princeton, New Jersey.

future members. However, they assumed these prerogatives slowly. Although the American Medical Association was founded in 1849 with education as one of its concerns, it was not until the 1890s that it was able to do much with regard to establishing educational standards, and it was not until after 1910 that there was really an effective programme of surveillance over education.

Having pointed out a few of the social factors that helped to fashion the methods of controlling educational standards in the USA, I shall now present several definitions of terms. The term 'credentialing' is now being used by some people as an all-inclusive term to apply to accreditation, certification, and licensure.

Accreditation is the process by which an agency or organization evaluates and recognizes a programme of study or an institution as meeting certain predetermined qualifications or standards. It applies only to institutions and their programmes of study or their services, and we generally use this term to apply to non-governmental agencies.

Certification is a process by which a non-governmental agency or association grants recognition to an individual who has met certain predetermined qualifications specified by that agency or association.

Licensure, which is a state function, is the process by which an agency of government grants permission to persons meeting predetermined qualifications to engage in a given occupation and/or to use a particular title, or grants permission to institutions to perform specified functions.

There is one other term which I add simply for clarification. *Registration* is the process by which qualified individuals are listed on an official roster maintained by a governmental or non-governmental agency. In some cases it is a synonym for certification or for licensure.

Accreditation has generally been conducted by associations of educational institutions by visiting, evaluating, and then listing for public recognition those institutions which have been considered to have met predetermined qualifications; and it is generally done on a non-governmental enforcement basis. We use the term 'voluntary' to apply to accreditation, but I insist that the use of this term is misleading, because there are social and indirect legal pressures which require that an institution attain accreditation in order to gain other benefits, such as financial grants from the Federal Government.

One additional point on accreditation. Accreditation is also conducted as a means of surveillance over programmes of study preparing individuals to enter many of the professions, especially the health professions.

Certification is conducted by non-governmental organizations to identify individuals, not programmes of study, but individuals who are considered to have met predetermined qualifications through the use of written, oral, or other tests, or other examining processes, to verify their competence to be considered certified or qualified individuals.

Licensure is the legal governmental responsibility of approving an individual to practise a profession. And this, in the USA, as has already

132

been indicated, is a responsibility of each of the 50 states. This factor of 50 separate legal jurisdictions creates various difficulties to which I will not draw your attention at this time.

Now, let me briefly point out some of the social factors which I contend are hindering us in providing adequate health care to many segments of our society, even though to the rest of the world we are the most affluent of people.

As has been the case throughout the world, we in the USA have been confronted with very definite population growth. We have had a concurrent growth in the number of educational institutions and in their variety. We have had an increasingly higher percentage of our population enrolled in educational institutions. And we have relied increasingly upon educational institutions to provide a major part of the education of individuals who are entering one of the health professions. These factors have increased the necessity to specify the institutions and programmes of study that have attained reasonable quality.

At the same time, a larger segment of the population has become fully cognizant of social, scientific, and professional issues. As we are all aware, there have been marked scientific and technological developments that are leading to and forcing greater interprofessional interdependence. There has been an increasingly active interest on the part of students in the education offered them, and students are no longer accepting without question the prescriptions that faculty in the past have assumed would be accepted without question. We have seen a greatly increased involvement of both the Federal Government and state governments in the delivery of health care.

As a result of many of these developments, we have had a fractionalization of health personnel into groups who are increasingly expressing their concern about the economic benefits that their members may receive.

Now, I shall turn to an issue which, to me, has very definite and broad social importance. I am referring to conflicts of interest, both actual and potential, between the welfare of professions and the welfare of society. The following outline may help to clarify my point.

Some concerns of professional associations:

1. *Social benefits*
   Educational
   Ethical standards
   Professional competence
   Scientific developments
2. *Personal benefits*
   Economic
   Political
   Social (including hierarchical)

We have too uncritically accepted the professions as defined by sociologists as being primarily interested in the welfare of society and only incidentally concerned with the benefits to their members. Interest in the welfare of society has been demonstrated by concern with the standards of the educational programmes of individuals being trained to enter the profession, concern with ethical standards, concern with the professional competence of those entering the profession, and now an increasing concern with the professional competence of those continuing to provide health care, as well as concern with scientific development. We have assumed that these were the only prerogatives of a profession and that all others were incidental.

Take the example of ethical standards. In what I am saying I wish to be constructively critical. A profession, to be considered a profession, is expected to develop a statement of ethics. This should continue to be the case. However, we must realize that the members of a profession will act in the same way as any other group of humans and look at their statement of ethics in terms of what will benefit the members of that particular profession, even though they will assume their ethics are purely for the benefit of society.

Let us turn to other concerns of professional societies with particular reference to the situation in the USA. With the growth of population and other social and economic developments, there is among the various professions a struggle for economic benefits, political status, and individual social status. This last includes hierarchical relationships, which are sometimes called the pecking order.

It is my contention that the social benefits of a profession, as listed above, should continue to receive the constant attention of its members. On the other hand, I have observed that because of various social forces, the professions are regretfully having to give more and more attention to the economic, political, and social welfare of their members, sometimes to the detriment of their concerns for the broader welfare of society. This observation is related to the subject of my talk in the following way—since the professions have a concern and a responsibility for conducting the accreditation and the approval of the educational programmes that prepare their future members for entry into the profession, their concern with their member's economic, political, and social benefits leads to the definite possibility of a conflict of interest with their professional concern for the benefit of society.

In accreditation, as I have indicated, the professions are largely responsible for the approval of the educational programmes; and in view of the social development of this country, it is logical that they should have that responsibility. It is also understandable that they possess the greatest concentration of professional and technical competence to exercise it. At the same time, since accreditation does have an indirect influence on the entry, it is my contention that there has to be a much greater broadening of professional responsibility than has developed in the USA up to the present.

Let me give you an example. During the past two days there has been repeated reference to the physician's assistant, associate, MEDEX—whatever term may be used. We have heard repeatedly the phrase that he or she is hired or employed by the physician.

This implies an initial assumption that there is a hierarchical relationship. More important to my contention, it connotes an employment relationship in which the physician's assistant is not only subordinate to the physician in the case of responsibility but is subordinate to the physician economically.

The USA now has strong labour unions, and we can no longer visualize employers controlling labour unions as might have been possible 50 or 75 years ago. My further point is that the terminology that you are using is an example of issues which may arise to haunt you in the future. It is my contention that the physician's assistant should be considered a colleague, one of the colleagues of the physician. I am not stating that the physician's assistant should be considered as having the same competence to practise as the physician. On the other hand, in a nation in which medicine belies the trend but continues to place emphasis on the entrepreneurial type of practice in which the physician wishes to consider himself as an independent practitioner, it is improper, in fact, it is injudicious, to speak of the physician's assistant as his employee with all that this term connotes.

Let us now return to the subject of accreditation. The American Medical Association (AMA) conducts a programme of accreditation for schools of medicine in collaboration with the Association of American Medical Colleges. In addition, it is involved in the accreditation of a number of allied health educational programmes. In the middle 1930s the AMA, following separate requests from the American Occupational Therapy Association and the American Physical Therapy Association, agreed to collaborate with those associations in the accreditation of programmes in occupational and physical therapy.

This development has now led to the point, as you heard from Dr Malcolm Todd, that there are approximately 22 fields accredited by the American Medical Association in collaboration with the groups preparing individuals as medical assistants, medical laboratory personnel, medical records personnel, nuclear medical personnel, occupational therapists, physical therapists, physician's assistants (including specialties which I am not mentioning individually), radiological personnel, and respiratory therapists.

In addition, there are fields in which individuals are prepared for various activities related to the delivery of health care, where accreditation of educational programmes is conducted without relation to the AMA: clinical pastors, community health, dentistry and dental auxiliaries, environmental engineering, hospital administration, nurse anaesthetists, nurse midwives, nursing, optometry, osteopathic medicine, pharmacy, podiatry, psychology, public health, social work, speech pathology, and veterinary medicine.

I have mentioned these simply to give you a panoramic view of accreditation in the USA; I shall conclude with a couple of observations.

Much has been said in the press recently of the undue attempt at concentration of power by a segment of our governmental force, and this concentration of power has led to misinterpretations of what is best for society. My concern is that the profession of medicine, on which the future of society relies for its health and its well-being, could unconsciously and unintentionally arrogate to itself more authority than would be good either for medicine or for society. As you consider these medical assistant programmes, I urge you to recognize that most of the individuals in this room are physicians. Even though we come from different backgrounds and face different social problems, nevertheless others than physicians must be included in the process of defining and delivering health care, and in that of developing and defining any new health profession, even when in the delivery of health it is subordinate to medicine.

My concluding statement is that we in the USA have not yet recognized the undue concentration of power in matters of accreditation that is now happening. Until we do, we continue to run the risk of upsetting unduly the balance of forces in our society, the balance of forces which was established by the Constitution, not only among the various branches of the Federal Government and between the Federal and state governments, but between government and the private sector.

LEGAL ASPECTS

by BLAIR SADLER, J.D.[1]

In the short period of time at my disposal, I will not attempt to give you a detailed analysis of all the legal issues which are raised by a new kind of health worker such as the medical assistant. However, I will review some of the problems which are often expressed in legal terms and which may have some relevance to your countries.

In the last two days we have heard the views of people from various parts of the world. I would like to recall briefly some of those observations which involve legal considerations. Dr Estes, for example, emphasized the need for flexible development in practice and the need for flexible laws. Dr Silver discussed the difference between diagnosis and assessment, and the games we often play with those words.

Dr Smith commented on extending the reach of physicians versus substituting for physicians and remote supervised practices. Yet, in Canada and some other countries, it is clear that nurse practitioners or other types of physician's assistants seem to be 'substituting' for physicians.

Dr Todd noted that the keynote of the programmes in the USA has been their variety. We have had pleas, however, emphasizing the importance of innovation and flexibility for a concept which is still very definitely in an embryonic stage of development in the USA.

Dr Conant distinguished between medical and health models and referred to a grey area between certain practices of medicine and nursing.

Dr Selden has made us aware of the three basic interrelated concepts of accreditation, certification, and licensure. It must always be kept in mind that licensure is only one of these control and review mechanisms.

We have also heard much discussion about what is probably the most fundamental issue—independence, dependence, and interdependence, and the distinction that must be made between legal independence and functional independence. Basically, we are discussing the question of ultimate responsibility for one's acts in delivering health care.

We must recognize that we ask of the law a great number of very important things. We ask the law to protect the public. We ask it to protect

---

[1] Assistant Professor of Law, Yale University School of Medicine, New Haven, Connecticut.

against excessive delegation of medical practice to non-physicians. We ask the law to give us some mechanism for providing ultimate responsibility for the delivery of care, whether by physicians, the medical assistant, hospitals, or governments.

We also criticize the law in many cases, often justifiably, for not being flexible enough. We say that the law provides too many barriers to change. It does not allow us to experiment or to innovate. In asking the law to be flexible, we ask that it should not always look backward and that it should not be the last institution to change. Finally, we ask the law to provide remedies to individual members of the public when they are hurt, or aggrieved, or the victim of low-quality medical care.

In the USA the basic legal concepts are ones of definition of practice and standards of care. What is the practice of medicine? What is the practice of nursing?

Unfortunately, our definition of medicine is made at the state level— by 50 different states. Medicine is usually defined as follows: no one shall 'diagnose, treat, operate, or prescribe' except a licensed physician. The laws then refer to the various ways in which one becomes a licensed physician.

We know, however, that despite what the laws actually say, nurses for years have been making judgements and have been caring for patients in a variety of settings. Most people would say that they were really 'diagnosing' and 'treating' within certain limits, even if they were not operating or prescribing. Nurses employ some elements or forms of diagnosis in coronary care units, for example, or in public health nursing.

We have a concept in our law called 'custom and usage' on which we rely to avoid having to change the letter of the law to meet changing practice over time. This allows some kind of flexibility to be breathed into the law.

We also have a concept called standing orders, which you have heard referred to by Dr Estes, Dr Fenderson, and others. This permits physicians to define the terms of practice in certain settings and, therefore, to limit the amount of discretion exercised when certain parts of the practice of medicine are delegated to others.

These are the basic background concepts against which the emergence of the physician's assistant was tested in the late 1960s. As a result there has been an enormous amount of legal change in the last three years. Ultimately, when we trained new kinds of health professionals and significantly changed the function of existing health professionals such as nurses, we relied on custom and usage and did not change our medical practice acts in any way. In view of the fundamental and rapid changes which have occurred, such reliance on former custom and usage may be a weak position.

In the last three years, more than 30 states have modified their medical practice acts in a variety of ways. Some have simply amended their medical practice act to say that those acts or functions which a physician wishes to delegate to a physician assistant or nurse practitioner no longer violate the medical practice act. This provides great flexibility. It does not define the tasks, but it gives tremendous discretion to the individual physician and individual practice, and that is one of its greatest advantages.

On the other hand, others would argue that it might give too much flexibility and freedom for a physician to decide what parts of medicine can be delegated to someone working under his supervision. All these amendments require that such services be rendered under the supervision, control, and responsibility of the licensed physician. This means that not only is the medical assistant or physician's assistant legally responsible, but the physician is as well. This is not a new concept in American law. Physicians have long been responsible for acts of various health workers who work with them and for them.

Several other states have passed laws which not only give authority to practise parts of medicine to physician's assistants while under the supervision and control of physicians, but require that such persons be approved by the Board of Medical Examiners at the state level. The theory behind this is that we then get a board review of the type of training and background that the person has had: this allegedly gives better protection to the public and also protects against excessive delegation.

The problem is that these boards have tended to fall into one of the traps that we have heard described in the last few days, namely, reliance on educational credentials and educational background and not on the competence of the person to perform certain tasks. In some states, California particularly, regulations have been developed by these boards that are so detailed that they do not permit the needed flexibility. Indeed, supervision has been defined so narrowly that the physician has to be on the premises at all times and has to be virtually directly involved with all patients at all times—hardly the kind of definition that is consistent with the development of the decision-making medical assistants that we have been discussing. That, indeed, is one of the dangers of giving what, I submit, is excessive legal regulatory authority to certain boards.

Another problem with this approach is, as Dr Selden has mentioned, that of overall responsibility. These boards are entirely controlled and composed of physicians, without any representatives of nurses, hospital personnel, physician's assistants, or members of the public. It is questionable whether they are as responsive as they might be to some of these other concerns.

Other states have asked their medical examiner boards to look at job descriptions of what a physician's assistant would actually do and under what degrees of supervision, rather than rely too much on educational credentials.

In the case of nurse practitioners, additional problems are raised, for you must then ask: What is the practice of nursing? If a nurse is being given training to carry out additional functions, not only is there the question of the violation of the medical practice act, but also the nursing practice act. We have some further problems because, in many cases, our legal definitions of nursing have not been changed for years. Many of them are very vague and focus only on health counselling, health teaching, and health maintenance. In fact, the definition of nursing that was written in 1955 and recommended by the American Nursing Association ended the last sentence with 'None of the above shall include the authority to diagnose or prescribe.' So many of our states actually have a definition which would directly prohibit the kind of medical decision-making that nurses are being trained to do and are doing very well.

We are now seeing changes being made in our nurse practice acts in several states such as Idaho, Arizona, and New Hampshire. The acts are quite flexible in that they give the board of nursing, often jointly with the board of medicine, the authority to develop new areas where nurses can expand their function.

The New York law has received much publicity as a new definition of nursing. I do not think it is satisfactory because it still prohibits nurses from making any diagnosis or giving treatment of a medical nature.

The other major issue that arises is that of standards of care—of malpractice and possibly negligent acts of a medical assistant. The law has always been that a physician's assistant or nurse practitioner, when performing the kinds of procedures and acts he is trained to do, should be held to the same standard of care that the physician would be held to.

Much attention has been given to the possibility or likelihood that physician's assistants will somehow increase malpractice and that there will be frequent lawsuits.

I doubt this. The film which was shown to us portrayed a busy physician who talked about rushing from patient to patient and his difficulty in concentrating on the most difficult problems. He appeared generally harassed. If you substitute for this a well-trained and well-supervised medical assistant, all indicators would suggest less likelihood of bad medical practice, mistakes, negligence, and a lawsuit. Lawsuits generally arise from dissatisfied patients, patients who feel physicians did not give them enough time, were hostile or were harassed.

It seems to me that patient rapport should improve as a result of the productive use of physician's assistants. In fact, in the last three or four years, we have not had a rash of lawsuits involving physician's assistants. This is really a mythical issue.

It is very important at the present time to pass flexible laws which give a great deal of opportunity for innovation and experiment, but which are very specific in placing ultimate responsibility on the physician. There is, therefore, legal supervision, but not legal independence for these new practitioners.

At the same time, such flexibility permits a great deal of functional independence in terms of the actual acts that are performed. Legal supervision indeed may well be exercised at a distance of several miles through a variety of radio and television hook-ups and back-ups and through periodic visits, and does not always require the personal presence of the physician. These, I think, are the most important points to be made.

The major alternative we would have to legal dependence would therefore be a series of very specific laws which would define strictly what legally independent practitioners could do. This would be very restrictive and very limiting, I think.

Finally, what you will need to consider for your own countries are a series of trade-offs in terms of ultimate responsibility and control. How much responsibility and discretion in the end do you wish to give to individual physicians? How much discretion do you wish to give the physician, vis-à-vis health care institutions and the hospitals, in the responsibility for such new personnel? How much responsibility will the government have, whether a regional government or a national government, in ultimate control and responsibility for such physician's assistants?

Finally, you will need to consider very carefully the pressure for uniformity and standards in this area. Uniformity is easier, but may limit what I believe is a great need for flexibility and innovation. Until there are more data on the impact of different types of physician's assistants and the quality of care they render, I believe it is premature to develop in the law very specific types of restrictions on the kind of physician's assistants we should have and in precisely what settings they should practise.

DISCUSSION ON ASSURANCE OF QUALITY, COMPETENCE AND ACCOUNTABILITY

Chairman: RICHARD SMITH, M.D.[1]

SMITH (*USA*): Dr Selden's definitions of accreditation, certification, and licensure are critical not only to our discussion but to an understanding of the conceptual framework within which the medical assistant exists in the USA. Very possibly these have implications for other countries also.

In this session, we should discuss not only the presentations made by Dr Selden and Mr Sadler, but also any further points you may have regarding the subject of this conference.

I would like to initiate a discussion on the relationship of the medical assistant to the physician as it is viewed in the USA. Our concern is that the medical assistant should be under the supervision of the physician, whether the physician is in the immediate vicinity or miles away. Permitting the medical assistant to function at great distances from his supervising physician was the only way for us to effect a change in our health system that would extend and expand the delivery of care. Perhaps Dr Estes and Dr Silver, who have had experience in situations where the supervising physician has legal responsibility for medical assistants working at a distance, might wish to comment on this.

ESTES (*USA*): The areas in which we need the physician's assistant most are those where there are no physicians to supervise their activities directly. We must think of both the legal and the ethical aspects of the problem.

Most statutes pertaining to physician's assistants specify that there must be supervision, and therefore we must be able to prove that there is indeed supervision, that there is someone who is periodically looking at the care delivered, that the records are being reviewed, and that the techniques are approved.

From the ethical point of view, we must be certain that this assistant, who is working with us in a system of care, does indeed understand his own capabilities and limitations.

Within those legal and ethical bounds, we are colleagues, and we hope that we are working for the same end, which is a better health care system for the people concerned. Most good administrators and team leaders realize this. The person at the top of the administrative structure has certain responsibilities, but he knows that for the best results people must work as colleagues and share responsibility without having a hard and rigid hierarchy.

All of us are attempting to evolve compromises which will accomplish a degree of supervision within the limits imposed by our current legal system.

---

[1] University of Hawaii School of Medicine, Honolulu, Hawaii.

142

SILVER (*USA*): Much of what we are discussing really is not very pertinent for our overseas visitors because their problem is quite different from ours.

In the USA there has been too much emphasis on the physician having control, as well as supervision, of the physician's assistant. I am not sure that this is desirable; the competence of physicians varies enormously. I can foresee in the future that physicians who are less than competent and give poor supervision will be hiring various types of physician's assistants. This will cause a downgrading of the performance of the physician's assistant rather than its maintenance at a high level.

Controls are needed so that the physician's assistant regulates himself and is responsible for the degree and competence of the care he gives. Without that, there is a danger that the physician will hire a physician's assistant for the physician's own benefit, without adequately considering the public interest.

DU GAS (*Canada*): In the northern nurse programme in Canada, nurses function as physician substitutes in remote and isolated areas. The controls lie in the system of health care delivery. There are base hospitals, located in strategic positions, with medical staff and senior nursing personnel, and there are satellite nursing stations. The nurses in the satellite stations communicate with the base hospital through radio telephone, so that they can at any time consult with a physician or with their nursing supervisor. They can also send patients to the base hospital. In addition, physicians travel to the nursing stations at regular intervals.

In the matter of legal controls, we have not yet run into difficulty although these nurses do many things that would be considered to belong to medical practice in the southern parts of Canada. The nurses are Federal Government employees, and the Federal Government assumes the responsibility. A statement from the Justice Department covers the responsibility of nursing stations.

We now have six universities providing specific training programmes for nurses going into northern areas. The programmes are financed by the Federal Government. They provide four months of intensive clinical training which includes history taking, physical examination, emergency treatment, etc. The nurses diagnose and prescribe. It has been estimated that they can handle approximately 95% of the cases which come to the nursing stations.

TABIBZADEH (*Iran*): If you want to introduce a new profession in the health sector, it is preferable to have a law. Just a few years ago in Iran, we started to develop a rural midwives programme. A law was passed by Parliament. The law not only ensures greater competence and greater support to the profession, but it also increases career status because workers know they have good support; their place in the whole system has been recognized by law.

From time to time, auxiliaries working in rural areas have given a preventive drug on orders of a physician, a child has died, and the case has been taken into court. It has often taken as long as three to four months to convince the judge and the court that the auxiliary had been ordered to administer the drug by a physician or the Ministry of Health.

Therefore, it is important to have a law for these workers who must act virtually independently even though under distant supervision. This is especially true in developing areas where there will be no physician but there will be distant supervision by the health centre.

FLAHAULT (*WHO, Geneva*): It may at times have seemed that this conference has been too much focused on the American problem. In fact, the discussion has shown that some problems connected with physician's assistants in this country

143

can be compared to those found in developing countries with other types of medical assistants.

We have spoken, for instance, about the distance separating the physician from the medical assistant; that is a problem of autonomy and supervision.

Supervision is a concept which is somewhat opposed to the concept of distance. Dr Du Gas has shown how we can compensate or try to compensate for this disadvantage through the use of certain techniques which will ensure a certain degree of supervision. That can be true in both developed and developing countries.

In the USA, an impression may prevail that the physician's assistant is a means to expand the practice of the physician, and therefore to increase his income. In most developing countries, where physicians are less numerous and communication facilities, equipment, etc. are in short supply, the primary objective is not to bring in more income to the physician but rather to offer more services of an elementary, basic character to the population.

In the legal field, by an effort of imagination a way could perhaps be found to permit a certain degree of automony for physician's assistants. This is certainly a delicate matter, but something should be done, with the agreement of enlightened physicians, to adapt the legislation to the existing situation.

Another important question concerns the training of physicians. Once physician auxiliaries are trained, the practice of medicine changes and so the training of physicians must change. If the physician wishes to keep a pre-eminent place in the health team, his training should be adapted to new conditions.

In developing countries, the role of the physician is no longer just to care for individual patients, but also to organize and to supervise the work of his team. It may differ from the traditional role that we know in developed countries which do not make use of medical or physician's assistants.

SADLER (*USA*): Much of this can be viewed in terms of public reliance. Whom should the public ultimately rely upon for some standard of quality of care? Obviously, in any system, the medical assistant himself should be responsible for anything he does, and that is the case here. So there is that element of reliance.

Again, should reliance be placed primarily on a physician who will be ultimately responsible, or should it be placed on an institution, the team or workers, or the government?

GORIUP (*Algeria*): This discussion of legislation and standardization has been a very stimulating one. We do have serious problems in this area. Very often I have the occasion to observe that medical assistants do not know what they are supposed to be doing and what they should not be doing. They are told that they may prescribe and may treat patients. They may also feel that they are being reproached for so doing, and this creates a sentiment of frustration.

There is a contradiction between the fact that the medical assistant should depend on the doctor, and the fact that, in reality, he is asked to exercise a considerable degree of independence. One possible solution, as Dr Flahault mentioned, might lie in the manner of organization of a health team instead of having independent workers.

It is also difficult to see how, for example, a paediatric assistant can fully depend on a physician who sometimes may know less about the subject than the assistant.

In the developing countries, if we can give our medical assistants only a limited degree of independence from the physician in the strictly curative field, we must accord them a very high degree of independence in public health, preventive medicine, mother and child health, vaccinations, mass campaigns, and community work.

SOOPIKIAN (*Iran*): It is not clear to me how this training programme was developed in the USA prior to obtaining legal permission.

In our country accreditation of any training programme is through the Ministry of Education. First, permission is obtained from the Ministry of Education to establish a training institution to provide graduates who fit the needs of the country. Then, if they are to practise medicine in some remote areas, they need a special law, but a law established prior to training.

We had a law in our country when we trained our medical assistants. It was passed by the Parliament and was specifically intended for that group. It defined how they should be trained, for how many years, what degrees they could take, and what they could do. At that time the law stated that medical assistants had to work in rural areas and townships of not more than 10 000 population. Since this did not apply to urban areas, there were no difficulties with the medical association. But if we want to introduce a new law relating to urban areas, then we will have to work out with the medical association how medical assistants will work in urban areas and how they will help physicians. But our real problem is the rural area, not the urban area.

It is very interesting that in the USA universities started to train these people and then said how the system was going to work. I would like to hear how this happened.

SELDEN (*USA*): Dr Soopikian, let me reply to your question. The experience in the USA does not represent a necessarily suitable example for any of your countries. A majority of the educational institutions are now financed and supported by either state or federal funds or both. However, a large number of the post-secondary school institutions are chartered in their respective states as private rather than public institutions. They are free, therefore, to institute any new programme without prior approval. However, in certain professional fields, their graduates may not be eligible to practise unless they have graduated from an accredited programme. Public institutions were free to start programmes assuming the lesiglature had appropriated sufficient funds. In many states there are now state coordinating boards which attempt to reduce duplication and excessive proliferation of programmes.

SILVER (*USA*): I want to ask how many people come from countries where a physician's assistant working in a private setting will be a matter of any interest. In this country, we expect that a large number of physician's assistants just will not work with the private practitioners. Is that true anywhere else in the world?

BEAUSOLEIL (*Ghana*): The situation in Ghana is rather complex in that the law permits the nurse, whether she has had any additional training or not, to set up a clinic, but he or she must work under constant or intermittent supervision of a physician. On the other hand, the private physician can pick anybody he likes from the street, give him any training that he likes, and get this person to assist him in the provision of care for his patients. However, the medical assistants are all trained by the government and are employed in the public sector. Although they are required to work under supervision, invariably they work on their own for long periods without supervision of any kind, and therefore they tend to be very independent.

So we have a rather complex situation which I do not think exists elsewhere.

TADELLE (*Ethiopia*): The question of licensing and other legal considerations are not peculiar to the USA. For instance, the medical assistants in Ethiopia are not entitled to operate private clinics, but they are allowed to run rural drug shops particularly in areas without any health facility. However, this sort of outlet is not relevant to the MEDEX, and I am concerned about their future role. On the whole, it appears that it is the whole career of the medical assistants in the USA that is in question, and not simply the legal aspects of their practice.

Medical corpsmen are accepted by the Army, but not by society at large. This is, in my opinion, an obvious contradiction.

Another case in point is perhaps the tendency to consider the MEDEX as providers of service to minority groups, particularly those in the inner city ghettos. I have heard that people in the ghettos are eloquent in voicing their demands, and in this context they may prefer to have doctors.

SMITH (*USA*): Let me respond specifically to one part of your question pertaining to the limitation of the medical assistant only to the minorities, the disadvantaged, and the poorest segments of the population. It is not our intention that this category of personnel in the USA should be used to treat only one class or one group of people, for precisely the reasons that you have suggested.

TADELLE (*Ethiopia*): Please do not think that any criticism is intended by the following remark. In view of the acute physician shortage in developing countries, the rational thing is to utilize medical assistants to provide services for the needy rural population. If the same logic holds, despite the complexity of the problem in the USA, then the medical assistant would be the main provider of care for minority groups.

SADLER (*USA*): In some of the early models, the law was modified as the training programme was begun. This was the case in the MEDEX programme in the State of Washington. In other states, the law did not change until a couple of years later. In some states laws were passed before there were any training programmes at all. There has been such public interest and public demand for more health services that legislators were saying that they wanted physician's assistants or medical assistants in their state. They wanted to change the structure before such training existed.

In the USA, medical assistants cannot open their own independent clinics; they will be under some formal physician supervision.

The military–civilian issue is an interesting one. Indeed, one of the most appealing arguments for trying the MEDEX approach and the physician's assistant approach was precisely the point that you raised—that many returning corpsmen did not have such an outlet when they entered the system. They are now in a civilian law system which is quite different from the military law system.

BEAUSOLEIL (*Ghana*): One thing has been bothering me all along.

In the situation in Ghana the medical assistant is more a substitute for the physician than an assistant or an aid. Therefore, he can practise independently of the physician.

In the USA he is an assistant or aid to the physician and, therefore, he is not allowed to work independently of the physician. What happens when he loses his supervisor either through death or through the supervisor's moving to another area? Perhaps he lives in an area where he cannot find another supervisor, or he may be trained by a programme which is not acceptable in the next state. Then he must move his entire family to another area where his type of programme is acceptable.

These are problems that need to be examined carefully now before it is too late and the situation gets out of hand.

We are lucky not to be faced with this problem of the physician's assistant being restricted to work with the physician.

SIDEL (*USA*): To take us away from the USA for a moment, if I may, several of you asked me if I would expand on the comments that I made about the feldsher in the Soviet Union and the barefoot doctor in China.

I hope that the brevity of the remarks that I made yesterday about the feldsher did not lead you to believe that I am negative about the role of the feldsher in the Soviet Union. It has been a most valuable role. In great measure its value lies in the fact that the feldsher is an integral, defined part of a health care system. He fits very well into that system and strengthens it.

With regard to 'credentialing', throughout the Soviet Union, which covers one-sixth of the earth's surface, there are common regulations for the training and job descriptions of the feldsher. These were promulgated by the Ministry of Health in 1946 and, with a few modifications, are still in force. There is a common curriculum and common examinations for all graduating feldshers throughout the country. The feldsher has an extremely well-defined and well-controlled role.

On the other hand, a most important point to be made is that the feldsher's role has been changing. Dr Beausoleil has just distinguished between the role of the assistant as a substitute for the physician and his role as an assistant to the physician. In the Soviet Union in the 1920s and 1930s the feldsher was clearly used as a substitute for the physician. This is still true to a limited extent in some rural areas of the Soviet Union. For the most part, however, the role of the feldsher has now shifted from a substitute role to a complementary role; the feldsher, particularly in the cities, now acts as a technically trained aid to the physician. This flexibility, the ability to change the role to meet new needs, is an important factor in the success of the feldsher model.

The contrast between the role of the feldsher and that of the barefoot doctor in the People's Republic of China does not lie in a distinction between 'intermediate-level' personnel and 'lower-level' personnel. These terms reflect a hierarchy, whereas the difference is one of function rather than of status. The distinction is better stated by saying that feldsher-type personnel, like those trained in the programmes in the USA, are 'technically based,' whereas the barefoot doctor role is 'community-based'.

In China, the *chijiao yisheng*, literally translated as 'barefoot doctors,' wear shoes except when they are actually growing rice. The term implies that they remain peasants, that they remain part of the community they serve. They perform medical work part-time, and for the rest of the time they work in the fields together with their fellow peasants. They are trained locally. There are no national standards for their training, so far as one can see. There are no national regulations about the kinds of work they may do or may not do. The contrast is great compared with the pattern of training and employment of the feldsher. Perhaps most important of all, the barefoot doctors serve as a bridge between the traditional system of medical care, in which many of the Chinese people have faith, and the more modern system.

I want to conclude by saying that I hope in the next conference, to which Dr Dy referred yesterday, we will talk not only about the use of the community-based model, such as the barefoot doctor, in those countries that, we have been told, are training such workers—Mexico, Iran, and Brazil—but also about the need for such workers in the USA. Mr Bathke, for example, has referred to the need for community-based health care personnel to serve American Indians. Family health workers have been trained in the South Bronx of New York

147

City; they live in the neighbourhoods in which they work, which are largely populated by black people and by Spanish-speaking people. They serve as a most valuable bridge between the people in those neighbourhoods and the medical care system. There are many other areas in which such workers could be most important.

MOUTSOURIS (*Greece*): I have two brief comments. The first concerns what Dr Smith said to Mr Tadelle about medical assistants. In my country medical assistants will be restricted to a certain class of people, mostly living in the rural areas. It would be very difficult for people in larger towns and cities to accept this type of new profession, at least at the beginning.

My second comment is about the supervision of the medical assistants. That would be unavoidable, and I think it is the only way, at least in my country, for this new profession to function. We doctors are supervised, too, very often, and I doubt if people will accept medical assistants without close supervision, whether it is by the public health service, the social security service, or the doctor responsible for a certain area.

MINKOLA-NDOSIMAU (*Zaire*): In my country medical assistants and other paramedical personnel have existed for some time. But there are certain points to be emphasized regarding the legal and accreditation aspects.

All medical categories, whatever they may be, must first be recognized legally. There are laws that regulate the art of the medical profession. Before 1960, it was only the Ministry of Public Health that, after research and studies carried out by commissions, could propose the legal text covering the various categories. After 1964, in addition to the Department of Public Health which proposes the legal text and regulations, the Department of National Health must also control, verify, and supervise the programmes proposed in order to establish the levels of these various categories of personnel.

This is one of the specific points in Zaire. The paramedical personnel who have been trained overseas face certain difficulties in integration·because the training they had received was not recognized in our system. This means that at the very beginning, there is a legal recognition before the establishment of various categories. These categories have a certain ladder. At the very top of the ladder is the MD, who has complete freedom in his own profession. Then there are medical positions—the medical assistant, the nurse, and the assistant nurse. These are the categories that exist in the diagnostic field. They work as a team, each with well defined responsibilities, under the leadership of the physician.

As far as private practice is concerned, until 1960 only the physician had full freedom to exercise his profession; the other categories could not practise privately. Since 1960, there have been certain modifications, especially in the case of the nurse and the medical assistant who can exercise their professions, but only under the general supervision of a physician.

For instance, if a medical assistant wants to open a small practice, he cannot do so without the authorization of a physician, and the physician himself will have to define the type of activities that this nurse or this medical assistant is authorized to carry out.

In recent years, the officials of the government have had to restrict the number of private practices carried on by such intermediate-level personnel. Because some of these small practices were opened in urban areas instead of rural areas, responsible authorities had to ensure that they would be geographically distributed in an appropriate manner.

148

WATSON (*Papua New Guinea*): When I first heard of the Duke University programme, I thought: 'It will never work. The public in the USA is too litigation-minded.' In my own country, the standard applied is 'within the limits of his training and experience and the realities of his situation.' I do not know whether that is a legal definition, but it gives an idea of how the courts work. For example, some of our intermediate-level people work in places where contact with the outside world is by two-way radio and by air strip. The air strip might be clouded in for 48 hours. Or they may be on small islands, reached only by boat; storms can isolate them for days. So far the courts have been very flexible in their attitude. But in the USA, that kind of approach could lead to endless argument.

From the point of view of developing countries, the longer we can do without too much legality, the better.

Some speakers have suggested that a team approach may simplify the legal problem. I take it this means sharing responsibilities so that one specialist auxiliary can refer to an auxiliary specializing in another field. But consider the realities of the situation. Many communities in developing countries have no skilled health services at present. If they must wait until a team is ready (and that means not only the trained workers, but housing, facilities, and transport), in a situation of uncertain economy and changing priorities, many areas of 10 000 or more population will wait many years for a health service. In such situations, we need a single multipurpose person who can go in with a base grade team, largely untrained. Without him, we may not get a health service started at all.

HENRIQUEZ (*Chile*): We have had a programme of auxiliaries for a year and a half in my country. It is in an urban area under my supervision.

In Chile there is great geographical variation. Infant mortality rates in certain sectors reach a level of 180 to 200 per 1000. The physician–population ratio is 1 to 4000, although in certain areas there is only one physician for every 30 000 population. Very frequently those who are assigned to rural areas request transfers to the large cities. We are faced with many of the same 'urban versus rural' problems that confront the developing countries.

Therefore we felt compelled to begin using a rural health assistant, at an intermediate level, who could be trained in a short time. Persons are selected by their own communities. In a period of six month's internship, we give these assistants a very basic training with an opportunity, in time, to increase their knowledge in the field of medicine. We provide them with information on agriculture so that they may also develop food resources in their own environment.

We have already trained 70 rural health assistants, and by the end of the year we expect to have trained 250. Next near it will be a national programme, training 750 per year, so that by 1976 we hope to have 2500 trained rural health assistants.

EL HAKIM (*Sudan*): Our regime of training for the medical assistant is a fully organized system, but it definitely needs some legal basis. The law has been very flexible in the Sudan towards this category of health worker. Some periodic laws prevent the medical assistant from engaging in private practice, and some laws regulate his duties in the remote places where he has no physician help whatever.

These laws legalize the work of the medical assistant enrolled in government or national services. However, the rules and laws that govern his activities are not laws of delegation but usually are periodic laws which concern two aspects—

they specify his type of work and prevent him undertaking any form of private practice.

HARDIN (*Malaysia*): In Malaysia many of the situations described by Dr Watson still exist, especially in the State of Sarawak.

Today we still do not have specific legislation to govern the practice of medical assistants. They have been working strictly within the government services and, therefore, the government guarantees their protection.

Recently many of our retired medical assistants have been employed by private firms, e.g., in factories, logging camps, and so on, with our blessing. We now strongly believe that the time has come for us to introduce laws to control the employment of hospital assistants outside the public services. We already have specific legislation for the use of midwives and nurses in the private sector.

So this session has been very useful to me. All the problems that have been spelled out here are very relevant to our situation, and we will try to avoid these difficulties when we draw up our regulations in the near future.

RUTASITARA (*Tanzania*): In my country the medical assistants are recognized and accepted by the people only by convention. There is no provision in the present medical practice legislation defining their status and responsibilities. However, the Chief Medical Officer, or his authorized representative, can give blanket approval for certain people to render such medical assistance while in the service of the public, state, or voluntary agency medical organizations.

Medical assistants are supposed to work under the supervision of qualified medical personnel. However, it very often happens that some of the employing agencies do not have doctors to exercise even remote supervision. For other employing agencies which do have doctors for supervision, there is no law to enforce that supervision.

Under such circumstances medical assistants tend to be more and more independent in their day-to-day activities and more responsible for their actions. Malpractice actions are taken individually and are judged on their own merits, bearing in mind the limitations imposed on the medical assistants with regard to practising medicine. These limitations are always made known to them during their training.

In summary then, medical assistants in my country are given letters of approval to render defined medical help in recognized health organizations under physician supervision. They are not allowed to set up private practice.

NATHANIELS (*Togo*): Before saying a few words on this subject of the legal aspects of the practice of medicine by medical assistants, I would like to point out that, in the French system, schools of higher education are established only by the State. We do not have private universities as do the Anglo-Saxon and some other countries. We follow the French system which we inherited. Our school for medical assistants, for example, was created by law, by a decree of the Council of Ministers. So from the beginning to the end of their training, everything comes under the State. In other words, it is legally recognized by the State.

In France, nevertheless, the physician has always wanted to have the right to participate in the decisions of the State concerning his profession, which he considers a liberal and honourable one. In France, therefore, we have what we call the Order of Physicians, which comprises not only physicians but also a subsection for midwives. This is the only institution that can grant licences to practise medicine, and it has very strong prerogatives. It has the right to take disciplinary measures. It can even go so far, for example, as to forbid the practice of the profession in case of malpractice or serious problems.

We have precisely the French system in Togo and perhaps this is true in other countries which were formerly French colonies. We have an Association of Physicians and Midwives.

As I said earlier, our medical assistant school was designed for nurses and midwives, and since midwives are already a part of this Association of Physicians I do not think that for us in Togo there will be a major problem in admitting the medical assistant to the Association.

Medical assistants have their rights, and they know what they can and cannot do. In the training programme we have included forensic medicine and medical ethics, so that students should know from the beginning the rules which govern their profession.

I was very pleased to note that Dr Mahler said, among other things, that medical assistants render very valuable service and that they must be considered as equal colleagues.

BEAUSOLEIL (*Ghana*): I have a question for Mr Sadler. In my own country, although there is no legislation governing the training and utilization of the medical assistant, there is machinery within the civil service structure for taking disciplinary action against the health centre superintendent—our equivalent of the medical assistant—who commits an act of misconduct. Regardless of whether the charge is civil or criminal, proceedings are instituted against him. What is the system in the USA for taking disciplinary action against a physician's assistant who commits an act of misconduct?

SADLER (*USA*): A variety of things can happen. There is not an organized national group of physician's assistants, such as there is in nursing, for example. There is usually not a separate board at the state level such as there is in nursing and medicine. Disciplinary proceedings, therefore, are not yet clear or defined.

What would probably happen in such cases is that some combination of criminal sanctions could be brought to bear if physician's assistants violate the basic statute that allows them to practise. This is usually done through the State Board of Medical Examiners. I believe that in the majority of the states where the State Board of Medical Examiners has some control over the physician's assistant and the physician who hires him, the Board clearly has the authority to take disciplinary action as they would against a physician. This action might have the effect that he could no longer practise or that he would be suspended for a certain period of time.

Then a civil action could be brought by a patient who was harmed in some way.

And finally, there are associations of physician's assistants that might take some disciplinary action although they do not yet have statutory authority to do so.

In addition, the training programme of which he was a graduate might attempt to take some action against him.

SMITH (*USA*): Let me briefly answer two questions that have been raised.

First, some think that American physicians who employ physician's assistants do so in order to make additional money. It is difficult to convince the public that this is not the case. The necessary overhead, equipment, rental of space, and use of ancillary personnel, resulting from the employment of a physician's assistant, all amount to about the same overhead that a physician may himself incur. The physician assistant's salary does not quite come up to what a physician would be making. Therefore, the system is a savings when you consider what the output is.

151

Second, what happens when a medical assistant's supervisor dies or the team breaks up? We have had such experience with MEDEX, since nearly 24% of our MEDEX have moved from one physician to another. In the State of Washington a physician who has a MEDEX died. Interestingly enough, the presence of a MEDEX in the community has helped that community to attract a physician, although previously it had been unsuccessful in getting a physician for ten or twelve years.

We have attempted in this session to begin a discussion of the large framework within which the medical assistant operates in the United States. We clearly could do little more than scratch the surface. We are trying to do someting to improve the health care delivery system. And we have recognized what Dr Mahler eloquently portrayed as one of the few things that we can do immediately to have some positive effect on the health care delivery system, not only here in the USA and in other industrialized countries, but in countries which have few doctors and limited resources.

EPILOGUE

THE PRINCIPAL ACCOMPLISHMENTS OF PROGRAMMES

by *EDWIN F. ROSINSKI, Ph.D.*[1]

What I shall do is present a summary of what I have been able to cull from the discussions of the past two and a half days that might best be described as principal accomplishments in the training and utilization of medical assistants.

There are a great many such accomplishments, and I shall concentrate on those which were cited most often and which seem to have received the greatest emphasis. Even from the failures in the training and utilization of medical assistants, priceless lessons have been learned.

One of the principal accomplishments in planning for the training and use of medical assistants has been an acute awareness that programmes must relate to the socioeconomic and cultural factors of each nation. In developing training programmes for any new type of health workers, such as medical assistants, too often in the past there has been a tendency to ignore these factors.

Another principal accomplishment is the demonstration that, for medical assistants to contribute usefully to the improvement of health, they must fit into the country's health care system. Again, like the cultural and socioeconomic factors, an awareness of each country's health care system is of paramount importance, and a plan by which medical assistants fit into that health care system must be designed. These two accomplishments are extremely significant because in the past there has been a tendency to develop programmes for the training of new types of health workers *de novo*, paying little, if any, attention to how these health workers fit into the scheme of a nation's health plans.

The awareness that medical assistants can be trained in a number of settings is still another accomplishment. It has been demonstrated clearly that medical assistants can be trained in programmes that are located in medical schools, in university and community hospitals, in completely new institutions unrelated to medical schools, in nursing programmes and in many other settings. It has been established that there really is no set way in which to define the training milieu; there are various ways in which medical assistants can be trained.

---

[1] University of California School of Medicine, San Francisco, Calif.

155

A fourth accomplishment—and one that has been cited repeatedly—is that programmes for training medical assistants can be initiated in a shorter length of time than programmes for, say, the education of physicians. Not only can they be initiated in a shorter length of time, but the time spent in training a medical assistant to provide quality health services in considerably shorter than the time required in educating a physician.

Another major accomplishment is that by having a category of health worker such as a medical assistant, a health career has been provided for a number of individuals who otherwise might have been locked out from any such career. There are obviously a large number of individuals who do not meet the criteria for admission to a university medical school nor desire a medical education, but who can become valuable colleagues of physicians by serving as medical assistants. The possibility of a series of new careers in the health field has been created by the development of programmes for the training of medical assistants.

Another major accomplishment is the demonstrable fact that the health team can be enlarged and made more effective and productive by including the medical assistant. Indeed, in a number of countries—and this has been mentioned repeatedly—the medical assistant does function effectively as a leader of the health team.

From most of the experiences, there is reason to believe that, by and large, the public accepts the use of medical assistants as providers of health services. There often has been a reluctance to expedite the training and use of medical assistants because of the subjective impression that the public would reject the notion of a medical assistant or his equivalent as a provider of individual health services. Therefore, another major accomplishment has been our ability to substantiate the argument that, if the public is well informed about the role of the medical assistant, and if a plan of utilization is soundly developed, the public will then accept the medical assistant as still another health worker dedicated to providing quality health services.

Another principal accomplishment is the evidence that the medical profession is not an insurmountable barrier to the development and use of medical assistants. Again, if a well-designed programme is prepared and serious consideration is given to how the medical assistant will be used, the fear many critics have voiced through the years that the medical profession would unequivocally reject the concept of the medical assistant can be allayed. Obviously, there always will be a number of physicians who reject that concept, but this is not generally the case nor is it a major issue in most countries. Furthermore, it has been shown that if a well-conceived programme on the training and use of medical assistants is presented, the nursing profession can become a strong supporter rather than a severe critic of the effort.

Another principal accomplishment is seen in the evidence indicating that medical assistants can work in a variety of settings, such as community or regional hospitals, university hospitals, clinics, dispensaries, aid stations, and the like.

Another principal accomplishment made clear, especially to health planners, is that considerable planning has to take place before medical assistants are actually trained and functioning as practitioners. As health planners discuss and plan the creation of new types of health workers, or redefine the roles of existing health workers, they must consider these health workers in relation to job performance, and job performance, in turn, must relate to the health care system.

Still another principal accomplishment is that, through the effective utilization of medical assistants, the medical profession has begun to take a critical look at itself. It is evident that nations and communities cannot produce medical assistants and, at the same time, continue to produce physicians in the same traditional mode: to do so is economically unrealistic! A significant and far-reaching accomplishment brought about by the use of medical assistants is that the medical profession has been motivated toward considering a redefinition of the role of the physician.

An obvious accomplishment is that medical assistants increase the number of health personnel providing health services. This is probably the single most important factor that originally led to their use. By having an individual such as the medical assistant as part of the health team, not only is there an increase in the number of health personnel but an increase in the efficiency of the team as a whole.

These accomplishments together amount to two final major achievements. By having more health personnel and by increasing the efficiency of existing health personnel, the availability of medical services for all citizens has improved. And the final result of the use of medical assistants has been the increased quantity and improved quality of health care. Medical assistants have been instrumental in improving the quality of life, and this, indeed, is a most significant accomplishment.

Perhaps there might be, indeed there must be, better ways to improve the quality of health of any nation than through the training and use of medical assistants. Their initial use appeared to be an expedient, but in a number of countries it proved in fact to be a practical and enduring solution to the health manpower crisis.

A final note, This conference has given each of us an excellent opportunity and an excellent setting for exchanging ideas and for offering arguments and counterarguments on the training and use of medical assistants. It is through meetings such as this that we can fully benefit from each other's experience and work together toward solving our health manpower problems. As we meet, discuss, and share, it can only encourage us to pursue our goal of improving the quantity and quality of health care.

THE PRINCIPAL OBSTACLES AND PROBLEMS

by LEONARD D. FENNINGER, M.D.[1]

Before I talk about problems and obstacles, which might also be defined as mountains to climb and new regions to explore, let me make two observations that perhaps have been inherent in much of the discussion without being very clearly stated.

First, most of the fundamental decisions about medical care and health and much of the actual care are provided within families by nonprofessional people. Frequently, when we get into discussions about what various kinds of people with special training should do, we forget that no mother is ever sued for malpractice for taking a splinter out of her child's finger.

In defining limits of functions, one should recognize that large portions of care are given by people who are quite outside what we normally consider organized systems. But the education and understanding of this group—that is, the nonmedical, nonhealth professional or nonofficial health personnel—are of extreme importance in all aspects of the health of many people.

Although nursing has not been discussed in detail, it has been implicit in all these discussions that nurses have an enormous role in providing health care and have long functioned in many of the areas we have been discussing.

The relative importance of medical and health care in the lives of individuals and families in any society or any social organization, and the value of health and medical care to that society have been repeatedly stressed here. It is evident that different members of society perceive the value and importance of health and medical care quite differently.

The professional view of the professional health worker is obviously very different from the view of the individual, and the economist's view is, in turn, different from that of the health professional. The politician's view is different from both. When we talk about medical care and health care, we talk about a group of social and human needs and functions that are perceived quite differently by the different components of society.

[1] American Medical Association, Chicago, Illinois.

158

A most important problem is the degree to which personal freedom of choice can be permitted in the context of a more general social need. A number of people have alluded to this in different ways. Dr Rosinski has already referred to the importance of recognizing that cultural, geographical, human, and economic resources and differences are paramount considerations in dealing with the reorganization of care and in preparing the people who will provide it. A number of you have observed that the total context of the social fabric and the attitudes of the country ultimately determine who will be able to give care effectively and in what settings.

The important differences between short-term and long-term problems have frequently been mentioned. Some problems are foreseeable and some are unforeseeable. The foreseeable ones are sometimes, but not always, dealt with through planning. The unforeseeable ones cannot be. Therefore, it is necessary to have plans and arrangements flexible enough or sufficiently broad for modifications to be made in the system of education and the system of delivery of care as required to meet and solve unforeseen problems. Such problems may arise in the educational system, which obviously affects outcomes from the very day that a child enters school, or in the attitudes of educators or students or their families or in the relative importance that people attach to the significance of health and disease. In any case, there are a number of problems that, even with the best planning, are not recognized in advance and have to be dealt with at the time they arise. Therefore, no system should be so rigid and fixed that it cannot accommodate new evidence and new problems.

It has repeatedly been stated that all of these problems are of long duration and are associated with other social problems. They are expressed differently at different times, and they are approached differently in different nations or in different sections within one nation or among various population groups within the nation.

For example, there has been some discussion of a possible difference or distinction between medical care and health care. It seems to me that, when there are a limited number of trained people and a very large health problem, much of which lies in the segment of sanitation and public health, this difference is relatively small. As more and more of the problems of public health and sanitation are dealt with by engineers or other kinds of people in the society, then the differences between medical care, public health, and public health care emerge. The emphasis depends on the health problems a nation or a society faces at any given time.

Much discussion has been devoted to means of accommodating to multiple forces and the recognition that expectation is always greater than demand, that demand for services is always greater than need, and that the need for services is always greater than the resources available within the society at any given instant to meet those needs.

The process of accommodation to these multiple forces and factors that we are all going through is, I think, part of the discomfort that we all feel, and one of the major reasons why this has been an extremely important conference. The rates of change of these attitudes and forces are accelerating, and at any time of acceleration, those who have the responsibility to see to it that health care is provided find themselves much more uncomfortable than they do when the rate of change is slower. Part of our uncertainty is a reflection of the very rapid rate of change of expectation, desire, scientific advances, and social evolution.

I wish that the questions of levels—high level, intermediate level and low level—had not come into the discussion quite so much. It seems to me these very terms create difficulties in our efforts to meet the health needs of individuals and communities. We are talking about different functions that can be performed by different groups of people with different kinds of preparation and different kinds of experience, not levels of relative importance or who should control what. What we should be concerned with is an examination of the needs of individuals and communities, the functions which can be created to serve those needs, and the competence of people to carry out those functions. In other words, the judgement should be made of the value of the person's contribution to society on the basis of how he carries out his function, and less on whether he is A, B, C, D, E, F, or G in some hierarchy of undefined values.

One of the problems in dealing with health and medical care is that we tend to become hierarchical and structural; we tend to be anatomists at times when we should be physiologists. Part of the problem in planning and providing services has to do with the hierarchy that we tend to impose on health care and on our thinking about health care.

The availability of resources has again been a recurrent theme; the most important resource, obviously, includes the students, the teachers, the practitioners, the administrators, and the individual members of the public themselves. In other words, human beings are by far the most important resource. They create the institutions for education and training and for the provision of medical and health care. There is tremendous variation in both the kinds of resources and the quantity of resources among the nations represented at this conference. Therefore, each has sought to solve the problems related to resources—human, institutional, and economic—in different ways.

The limitation of financial resources and the problems that this creates, and questions related to the distribution of financial resources to health services as compared with other equally significant and imperious social needs in each nation have been discussed, but we have reached no conclusion.

In closing, let me mention some of the factors that seem to influence the decisions that have to be made about the allocation of resources of all types.

The first factor, as I have already mentioned, has to do with demand for health care as compared with need as compared with expectation. Great variations in demands, needs, and expectation exist among members of a single nation as well as among members of different nations. There are differences, for example, between a well-to-do urban group and a poor urban group, or a well-to-do urban group and a well-to-do rural group, or a poor urban group and a poor rural group. These differences in demand and expectation are related to differences in income and education.

Second, a factor which very strongly affects decisions is the degree of awareness that public and professional groups have of the differences between need and demand and the acceptance of responsibility on the part of the public and the professional groups for health care.

Third, the degree of understanding and acceptance of arrangements for health care strongly influences the allocation of resources. People have frequently mentioned that there is no system of medical care in the USA. Actually there are very well-defined systems of medical care that are quite rigidly codified. The problems lie in the fact that these systems of care do not meet the needs of the people who constitute society. There are two things that have to be done. One is to modify existing systems to correspond with changed needs. And the second is to be sure that people are prepared to fit within the existing system, to bring about the modification, and to participate in the modification as it inevitably takes place. Not only does the degree of understanding and acceptance of care influence the decisions on resource allocation, it also is a very significant factor in the preparation and the use of personnel.

Decisions on the quality as compared with the quantity of care are very important determinants in the allocation of resources, as are, of course, the economy of the country, its social and governmental organization, the degree to which government is centralized, and the degree to which responsibility is decentralized.

There has been a good deal of discussion of standards, and at times I have been a little confused as to whether it was standards or standardization that was being discussed. I think that there is a difference between the setting of standards and the standardization of programmes. Standards can be set on a much broader scale than one can standardize an educational programme or standardize a means of care or standardize functions, if standardization is to be uniformly and generally applied to large populations.

In addition to setting standards and determining who will set them, there is also the question of monitoring performance and maintaining standards. Legal systems and their variations in different nations strongly influence the kinds of decisions that are made about resources; similarly, political factors have become increasingly significant in all nations in the decisions about how resources will be allocated and who will benefit from programmes supported from public funds.

I hope in the brief discussion that is to follow some of the following questions will be asked:

The first is how to define the problems of health. Who is to make the definitions, and what kinds of limits and ranges are set? What services are needed to alleviate the inadequacies of health care in any given country?

Second, what ways have been tried of informing the people who ultimately decide on the allocation of resources for health services and medical care about the many factors involved in health and in health care so that they will anticipate the consequences of the decisions before finally making them? What ways have been found to help the public not only to understand what is happening but to take an interest in it and to contribute to the constructive development of health services?

What kinds of devices, tactics, and strategies can be used so that the various elements that are affected by health care and affect health care can be included early in the planning stage and can be involved in carrying out the care? There have been many allusions to physicians as conceiving of themselves as the sole providers of medical and health care.

In the discussion of teams, I think we have tended to talk about a sub-team when we have talked about the health professions. But the team ultimately includes the patient, the family, the industrialist, the politician, the economist, the administrator, and all of the other people who make up society. To some degree they are all involved in medical care and health services.

What experience have we had in altering the vested interests of educators, of administrators, of practitioners, and various organized groups? What experience have we had in influencing these groups to recognize that they ultimately serve and will continue to serve well only if they serve the public interest?

PITCAIRN (*USA*): At this point the session is open for general discussion or questions addressed to Dr Rosinski or Dr Fenninger.

BAKER (*USA*): There are two points that have not been covered extensively during the discussions although I believe them particularly important.

First, the point that Dr Flahault made in the initial presentation—that we should base all planning on the total population, in terms of numbers, distribution, and economic levels. This indeed guides us in setting the various levels and deciding on the numbers of health auxiliaries that are trained, and it focuses attention on the problems of distribution of health workers to meet the needs of populations. We must always look back to the population in planning because, indeed, this will set our objectives.

Second, there is a great need to exchange information on effective training methods, on techniques, at all levels. There are many new educational methods that have been used and that can be applied to this most difficult of all tasks, namely, to train a person with the smallest prerequisite education in the shortest time to fulfil what is potentially the most difficult job in the health sector.

THE FUTURE PROSPECT

by DANIEL FLAHAULT, M.D.[1]

Dr Rosinski and Dr Fenninger have summarized the discussions very well. May I just add a few concluding remarks.

First, we should remember that we should not, in any of our countries, attempt to economize on the services offered to the public. All our efforts should be based on this understanding. We should be aware that in many rural areas, even in a country such as the USA, health services are not always able to meet the demand and do not cover the entire population.

Another point of which we should be aware—and this is particularly important to those of us who deal with personnel training—is that our teaching programmes must constantly be reviewed. If we retain only one idea from this meeting, it is that we should constantly review the needs and the programmes established to meet these needs. We should not think that these programmes could be reviewed later, but we should begin to rethink them already now.

We must also resign ourselves to the fact that our ideals will never be realized, but that is no reason not to try to do something. This is simply common sense and perhaps sometimes common sense can be useful.

Another comment which is worth repeating is that we should admit that supplying even a limited service is better than no service at all. Personally, I believe it is better to be able to give something to a patient who has nothing. There are people who dispute this point, and that is one of the many obstacles to overcome in order to provide health services with medical assistant programmes.

I would like to mention four obstacles to change. I will simply list them briefly. The first probably is conservatism, the tendency of men and institutions to maintain the status quo. The second obstacle is bureaucracy. I believe that this exists in every country and in every international organization. The third is the complexity of change. It is always difficult to change and to revise what we are accustomed to. The fourth—and I do not think this is an exhaustive list—is the rapid diminution of resources in many countries. This is another major obstacle, but it should not discourage those who have the enthusiasm to work energetically for change.

---

[1] World Health Organization, Geneva, Switzerland.

What are the prospects for the medical assistant in the future? To reply to this question, we must first examine the needs and the means. The needs and the requirements of the community and of society have frequently been discussed during the conference. They are qualitative and quantitative. There are certain priorities which must be established. Problems of coverage come before problems such as the different kinds of service.

Then there are the requirements of the services themselves, services which, in many countries are financed by governments with limited resources. A very good formula can be summarized as follows: We must have the maximum of services in a minimum amount of time for the maximum number of people. This is a problem of economic efficiency and therefore of planning.

What are the needs of health service personnel? They must perhaps have more interesting work, a better life. Doubtless these concerns should be taken into account. This leads to the idea of teamwork that many of you have stressed, and the idea of the different levels of health workers and the way they are distributed.

We have different kinds of teams in different countries, and we have heard different ideas expressed here. It has been said that there are multiple forms of medical assistants, that these teams vary from one individual to an entire series of teams and subteams.

In addition to these needs, there are undoubtedly certain constraints related to society. There is a problem in demographic growth, and this means that requirements will increase, society will develop, and needs are going to grow; there will be increased demands even though resources will remain limited.

Another constraint is lack of personnel, and this will become increasingly acute because of the working conditions. Personnel will demand more with respect to working conditions and living standards.

Can we count on an increase of resources and an increase of available financing within a country? Unexpected things can happen. For example, we have seen in the past decade the case of Libya, a country that has obtained resources enabling it to develop much more rapidly than was originally foreseen. However, it is not always possible to count on such miracles. Experience shows that we must count on ourselves, particularly, and count much less on other people or on external resources.

The growth of resources and personnel, more physicians, more nurses, more technicians, in various fields—this is certainly a goal but is it a solution? Probably not. I can give you an example that I came to know about when I was in Russia.

In the Caucasus, for 10 000 inhabitants in a very rural area there were 14 physicians. This is an excellent figure for a rural area. But in a region the size of Belgium, these 14 physicians were all concentrated in a single hospital, and had no contact with the people except through the feldshers. There was an increase in physicians if the hospital was enlarged, but there was no increase in physicians available to the population. Even a socialized country like the Soviet Union did everything possible to bring physicians to places where living and working conditions were better than in an isolated rural area.

Assistance in personnel from international aid, bilateral assistance, is only a stopgap. It is only a provisional, temporary solution: it cannot be the answer. We need to find this answer in our own countries. Yet the development of any infrastructure depends upon an increase in means and in personnel.

Dr Mahler has said that we should try to be rational in an irrational world. It is very likely that this should be our first step—to try to be rational, to try to use our means to the best effect, and to try to determine who is to do what. These are problems of task analysis: determine the definition and composition of health teams, determine action priorities, establish the objectives of our teaching programmes, establish the teaching programmes themselves and adapt them to our task.

I am not telling you anything new. This is a problem of planning teaching and instruction and of how to train teachers. Perhaps during this session we have not sufficiently stressed the need to train teachers to work with these personnel, to prepare manuals, and to assess, review, and revise our programmes.

Therefore, to be rational in our use of means, we must ensure that supervision is organized and institutionalized, without, however, waiting until the entire structure has been created. We must bear in mind what Dr Rosinski said about the need to review physician training and to make physicians aware of their role in supervision and organization, a role that they must play as head of the team.

When we work in underdeveloped or developing countries we sometimes have a tendency to try to go too fast. However, we should adapt ourselves to the rate of development of the country. There must be a certain equilibrium in development. We cannot develop health services more rapidly than the rest of the country's services are developing.

One last point to be stressed concerning the developing countries is the need to give our health personnel a sense of responsibility in the development of the country. It goes without saying that health service personnel are there to develop health services, but they should also realize their role both in the development of the community and in the development of the country. Health personnel placed in a peripheral point where they most often work with the local teachers, the priest, the pastor, people who have a certain level of education, the most eminent people of the region—at this point, they have a role to play in developing the country, and they must be made aware of this role. Their aspirations and actions should not be limited to health services. They must be able to advise the local authorities in matters of economic development, agricultural development, village development, and sanitation. All of these are basic functions that are sometimes forgotten in training programmes.

As for the future in the developed countries, the problem is undoubtedly primarily a qualitative one. We have taken care of the basic needs, but we need to improve the nature, the number, and the quality of services offered. We must, of course, consider improving the working and living conditions and the quality of life of the physician as well as the other health personnel.

In the developed countries, the problems are less dramatic; these countries have financial and personnel resources which make it possible for them to bear the burden, and provide the effort necessary for the country's development. The developed countries, the developing countries—these are very temporary distinctions and all the developing countries are called upon to become developed countries.

What does the future hold in this area? Perhaps the progress of certain countries may be taken as a model. We can draw lessons from the recent history of Europe. In the last century there were medical assistants with different names in different countries. This category of personnel has now disappeared, and its functions have been distributed among physicians, nurses, and other personnel, yet we cannot say that the solution adopted was the best one.

In the Soviet Union, it is interesting to note the evolution of the role played by the feldshers. Dr Sidel reminded us of it. At the time of the revolution of 1917, the USSR had a tremendous lack of physicians and found in the feldshers a means to bring certain services rapidly to the people and, particularly, to the rural populations. At that point the feldshers played a role in which they substituted for physicians.

Now, some 55 years later, the USSR continues to train as many physicians as it trains feldshers, and it trains about 30 000 feldshers per year. But the feldshers of 1973 have little in common with the feldshers of 1917. Their role has become much more one of assistance and sometimes a more specialized one.

I do not want to pursue this point. Many articles have been published on it. But I would simply like to remark that, in all countries that are training this kind of personnel, there are possibilities for changing their role if some day it is found that there are too many of them in a given area. And I think the example of the USSR is a quite valid one.

In conclusion, I would simply like to recall what we said at the beginning of this conference, that the medical assistant is certainly not a final answer. It is a means among others to improve health services, and it is a means which has not been sufficiently exploited. It could be used to much greater advantage if the problem of the medical assistant were envisaged objectively and without prejudice. I do not want to make any distinctions between the various roles and functions of the medical assistant, but I think that some form or other of the medical assistant, whether it be at a central level or completely at the periphery, can be adapted to the conditions of any given country.

———

BIBLIOGRAPHY

American Medical Association, Department of Manpower Intelligence & Bureau of Health Manpower Education, National Institutes of Health (1972) *Summary of training programs; physician support personnel*, Washington, D.C., Department of Health, Education, and Welfare (Publication No. NIH 73-318).

American Medical Association, Council on Health Manpower (1972) *Guidelines for development of new health occupations*, Chicago, Ill.

American Medical Association (1972) *Status and utilization of expanding and emerging health professions in hospitals*, Chicago, Ill.

Bates, B. (1970) Doctor and nurse: changing roles and relations. *New Engl. J. Med.*, **286**, 129–134.

Bryant, J. (1969) *Health and the developing world*, Ithaca, Cornell University Press.

Denison, J. D. (1968) Physician assistants: a threat or a challenge? *J. Maine med. Ass.*, **59**, 224–225.

Estes, E. H., Jr. (1970) The training of physicians' assistants: a new challenge for medical education. *Mod. Med. (Minneapolis)*, **38**, 90–93.

Fendall, N. R. E. (1972) *Auxiliaries in health care; programs in developing countries*, Baltimore & London, published for the Josiah Macy Jr Foundation by the Johns Hopkins Press.

Fendall, N. R. E. (1972) Auxiliaries and primary medical care. *Bull. N.Y. Acad. Med.*, **48**, 1291–1300.

Flahault, D. (1972) The case for medical assistants. *Wld Hlth*, June, pp. 8–15.

Flahault, D. (1972) The training of rural health personnel. *WHO Chronicle*, **26**, 243–249.

Gish, O., ed. (1971) *Health manpower and the medical auxiliary*, London, Intermediate Technology Development Group.

Gordon, I., ed. (1971) *World health manpower shortage: 1971–2000*, Durban, Butterworth.

King, M., ed. (1966) *Medical care in developing countries. A primer on the medicine of poverty and a symposium from Makerere*, Nairobi, Oxford University Press.

Lippard, V. W. & Purcell, E. F., ed. (1973) *Intermediate-level health practitioners: report of a Macy conference on intermediate-level health personnel in the delivery of direct health services*, New York, N.Y., Josiah Macy Jr Foundation.

Morgan, R. H. (1968) Physician assistants: their role in medicine in the years ahead. *J. Maine med. Ass.*, **59**, 219–223.

Nurse practitioners. *Hospitals*, 1970, **44**, No. 9, 56–57.

Rifkin, S. B. (1972) Health care for rural areas. In: Quinn, J. R., ed. (1972) *Medicine and public health in the People's Republic of China*, Bethesda, Md, Fogarty International Center, US Department of Health, Education, and Welfare, pp. 137–149.

Rosinski, E. F. & Spencer, F. J. (1965) *The assistant medical officer*, Chapel Hill, University of North Carolina Press.

Rosinski, E. F. & Spencer, F. J. (1967) The training and duties of the medical auxiliary known as the assistant medical officer. *Amer. J. publ. Hlth*, **57**, 1663–1669.

Sadler, A. M., Jr et al. (1972) *The physician's assistant: today and tomorrow*, New Haven, Yale University Press.

Sidel, V. W. (1968) Feldshers and 'feldsherism': the role and training of the feldsher in the USSR. *New Engl. J. Med.*, **278**, 934–939, 987–992.

Sidel, V. W. (1972) Medical personnel and their training. In: Quinn, J. R., ed. (1972) *Medicine and public health in the People's Republic of China*, Bethesda, Md, Fogarty International Center, US Department of Health, Education, and Welfare, pp. 151–171.

Smith, R. A. (1969) Medex: a demonstration program in primary medical care. *Northw. Med. (Seattle)*, **68**, 1023–1030.

Todd, M. C., & Foy, D. F. The current status of the physician's assistant and related issues. *J. Amer. med. Ass.*, **220**, 1714–1720.

WHO Expert Committee on Professional and Technical Education of Medical and Auxiliary Personnel (1968) *Training of medical assistants and similar personnel; seventeenth report of the . . .*, Geneva (*Wld Hlth Org. techn. Rep. Ser.* No. 385).

World Health Organization (1973) *Suggested guidelines for planning, implementing and evaluating a programme for the training and use of medical assistants* (Document No. 2 on the use of 'medical assistants' for improving health services), unpublished document WHO/Educ/73.164 (available on request from the Division of Health Manpower Development, World Health Organization, Geneva).

The training and utilization of feldshers in the USSR. *WHO Chronicle*, 1972, **26**, 299–301.

Annex

LIST OF PARTICIPANTS[1]

Dr Héctor R. Acuña, Director General, International Affairs, Secretaria de Salubridad y Asistencia, Mexico 5 D.F., Mexico.

Mr Jerry Bathke, Executive Director, Navajo Health Authority, Window Rock, Arizona.

Dr Edwin G. Beausoleil, Deputy Director of Medical Services, Ministry of Health, Accra, Ghana.

Dr Propicio Caldas Filho, Secretary of Health, Government of the State of Paraíba, Av. Pedro I, SIN, João Pessoa, Brazil.

Dr Lucy Conant, Dean, School of Nursing, Carrington Hall, University of North Carolina, Chapel Hill, North Carolina.

Dr Tran-Tri Dien, Chargé de Mission, Ministère de la Santé, 59 Hong-Thap Tu, Saigon, Viet-Nam.

Dr P. Diesh, Director General, Health Services, New Delhi, India.

Dr Beverley M. Du Gas, Chief, Health Manpower Planning Division, Health Manpower Directorate, Ministry of National Health & Welfare, Ottawa, Ontario, Canada.

Dr E. Harvey Estes, Jr, Professor and Chairman, Department of Community Health Sciences, Duke University School of Medicine, Durham, North Carolina.

Dr Douglas Fenderson, Director, Office of Special Program, Bureau of Health Manpower Education,[2] National Institutes of Health, Bethesda, Maryland; Director, Continuing Medical Education, University of Minnesota, Minneapolis, Minnesota.

Dr Leonard D. Fenninger, Director of Graduate Education, American Medical Association, Chicago, Illinois.

Professor Malcolm A. Fernando, Department of Preventive and Social Medicine, Faculty of Medicine, University of Ceylon, Peradeniya, Sri Lanka.

Dr Daniel Flahault, Chief Medical Officer for Training of Auxiliary Personnel, Division of Health Manpower Development, World Health Organization, Geneva, Switzerland.

Dr Sobhi Y. El Hakim, Assistant Under-Secretary (Training), Ministry of Health, Khartoum, Sudan.

Dr Stalin Hardin, Acting Assistant Director, Medical Services, Medical and Health Office, Kuching, Sarawak, Malaysia.

Mr Thomas Hatch, Director, Division of Allied Health Manpower, Bureau of Health Manpower Education,[2] National Institutes of Health, Bethesda, Maryland.

Dr Hernán Henriquez,[3] Director de Zona, Servicio Nacional de Salud, X Zona de Salud, Calle Prat 020, Temuco, Chile.

---

[1] Affiliations and titles shown are those as of the date of the Conference. New affiliations are shown in italics.
[2] *Now* Bureau of Health Resources Development, Health Resources Administration.
[3] Since deceased.

Dr Abraham Horwitz, Director, Pan American Sanitary Bureau, WHO Regional Office for the Americas, Washington, D.C.

Dr Milo D. Leavitt, Jr, Director, Fogarty International Center, National Institutes of Health, Bethesda, Maryland.

Dr Halfdan T. Mahler, Director-General, World Health Organization, Geneva, Switzerland.

Mr Tadelle Mengesha, Chief, Planning Division, Ministry of Public Health, Addis Ababa, Ethiopia.

Dr Nkondi Minkola-Ndosimau, Director-General, Department of Public Health, Kinshasa, Zaire.

Dr Christopher Moutsouris, Associate Professor, Second Department of Propedeutic Surgery, Athens University School of Medicine, King Paul Hospital, Athens, Greece.

Dr Emmanuel Nathaniels, Director, Medical Assistants School, University of Benin, Lomé, Togo.

Dr Donald M. Pitcairn, Special Assistant of the Director, Fogarty International Center, National Institutes of Health, Bethesda, Maryland.

Dr Edwin C. Rosinski, Professor of Health Sciences Education, University of California School of Medicine, San Francisco, California.

Dr William Rutasitara, Senior Medical Officer, Preventive Services Section, Ministry of Health, Dar Es Salaam, Tanzania.

Mr Blair Sadler, Assistant Professor of Law, Yale University School of Medicine, New Haven, Connecticut; Assistant Vice President, Robert Wood Johnson Foundation, Princeton, New Jersey.

Dr William K. Selden, Immediate Past Director, National Commission on Accrediting, Princeton, New Jersey.

Dr Victor W. Sidel, Chief, Department of Social Medicine, Montefiore Hospital, Bronx, New York.

Dr Henry K. Silver, Professor of Pediatrics, University of Colorado Medical Center, Denver, Colorado.

Dr Richard Smith, Office of the Dean, University of Hawaii School of Medicine, Honolulu, Hawaii.

Dr George Soopikian, Director General of Planning, General Department of the Planning of Health, Ministry of Health, Teheran, Iran.

Dr Iradj Tabibzadeh, Director General, Malaria Eradication Organization, Ministry of Health, Teheran, Iran.

Dr Malcolm C. Todd, Chairman, Council on Health Manpower, American Medical Association, Chicago, Illinois.

Dr Manasvi Unhanand, Deputy Under-Secretary of State, Ministry of Health, Bangkok, Thailand.

Dr Ramon Villarreal, Chief, Department of Human Resources, Pan American Health Organization, Washington, D.C.

Dr Ernest J. Watson, Principal, Paramedical Training College, Department of Public Health, Yomba, Madang, Papua New Guinea.

OFFICIAL OBSERVERS

Dr Timothy D. Baker, Department of International Health, School of Hygiene and Public Health, Johns Hopkins University, Baltimore, Maryland.

Dr George Blue Spruce, Bureau of Health Manpower Education,[1] National Institutes of Health, Bethesda, Maryland.

Dr Thomas D. Dublin, Office of the Director, Bureau of Health Manpower Education,[1] National Institutes of Health, Bethesda, Maryland.

Dr Francisco J. Dy, Regional Director for the Western Pacific, World Health Organization, Manila, Philippines.

---

[1] *Now* Bureau of Health Resources Development, Health Resources Administration.

Dr Hassan Fateh, Associate Professor, Radiology Department, Teheran University, Teheran, Iran.

Dr Sergio Goriup, World Health Organization, BP 142, Constantine, Algeria.

Dr Isaiah A. Jackson, Jr, Embassy of the United States, U.S. Agency for International Development, Saigon, Viet-Nam.

Dr Roger LeClercq, World Health Organization, P.O. Box 343, Vientiane, Laos.

Ms Florence Reynolds, Inter-Organization Relations Office, National Center for Health Services, Research and Development, Health Services Mental Health Administration,[1] Rockville, Maryland.

Ms Jessie M. Scott, Assistant Surgeon General, Director, Division of Nursing, Bureau of Health Manpower Education,[2] National Institutes of Health, Bethesda, Maryland.

Dr Emanuel Suter, Director, Division of International Medical Education, Association of American Medical Colleges, Washington, D.C.

---

[1] *Now* Health Services Administration.
[2] *Now* Bureau of Health Resources Development, Health Resources Administration.

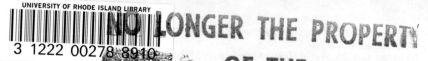
PUBLIC HEALTH PAPERS